A
YEAR
OF
NOTHING

**Also by
Emma Gannon:**

Fiction:
Olive
Table for One

Non-fiction:
Ctrl Alt Delete
The Multi-Hyphen Method
Sabotage
Disconnected
The Success Myth

Praise for
A YEAR OF NOTHING

'*A Year of Nothing* is a memoir, focusing on time spent doing nothing following a period of burnout: joys of slowing down, the beauty of cold water swimming, the power of slow news – and learning to say "no".'
– *Radio Times*

'Emma Gannon's honesty, open-mindedness and willingness to be vulnerable lays out a path for her readers to follow.' – Julia Cameron, author of *The Artist's Way*

'The new bible for thirty- to forty-year-olds.' – *ELLE Italy*

'[Gannon] is determined to carry the lessons from her burnout, and her recovery, into a slower, more spacious life.' – BBC Culture

'You might imagine that escaping from your everyday life would involve relocating to a Hebridean croft or attending a series of rejuvenating retreats. But, according to Emma Gannon's new book project, *A Year of Nothing*, it could be as simple as staying at home.' – *Guardian*

'Gannon explores what she learnt from her "burnout buffer".' – *ELLE UK*

'A book showing us how to recharge in smaller ways when taking time out isn't always possible.'
– BBC *Woman's Hour*

'A candid account of Gannon's descent into that year of profound loss of self, personal reckoning and reclamation.'
– *The Good Life Project Podcast*

Praise for
Emma Gannon

'If you're British and of a certain age, Emma Gannon will need no introduction. She is the Elizabeth Gilbert of the millennial age.' – Farrah Storr, author of *The Discomfort Zone*

'Emma is a guiding light for those who are driven to find purpose and fulfilment. She never fails to encourage me to take an unconventional path to a better way of living and working.' – Mo Gawdat, former Chief Business Officer of Google X

'I love Emma Gannon's wise and refreshing perspective on work and building a meaningful life.'
– Oliver Burkeman, author of *Four Thousand Weeks*

'A bright light and a shining star, and in many ways the voice of a generation.' – Elizabeth Gilbert, author of *Eat Pray Love* and *Big Magic*

A YEAR OF NOTHING

Emma Gannon

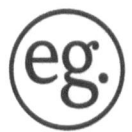

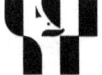

First edition published in 2024 by Emma Gannon,
in partnership with the Pound Project Limited

Revised edition published in 2026 by Emma Gannon,
in partnership with Whitefox Publishing Limited

www.emmagannon.co.uk
www.wearewhitefox.com

Copyright © Emma Gannon, 2024
Revised Edition Copyright © Emma Gannon, 2026

EU GPSR Authorised Representative
LOGOS EUROPE, 9 rue Nicolas Poussin, 17000, LA ROCHELLE, France
E-mail: Contact@logoseurope.eu

ISBN 978-1-9175235-8-5
Also available as an eBook
ISBN 978-1-9175235-9-2

Emma Gannon asserts the moral right to be identified as the author of this work.

All rights reserved. No part of this publication may be reproduced, stored in a retrieval system or transmitted in any form or by any means, electronic, mechanical, photocopying, recording or otherwise, without prior written permission of the author.

While every effort has been made to trace the owners of copyright material reproduced herein, the author would like to apologise for any omissions and will be pleased to incorporate missing acknowledgements in any future editions.

pp.58-59 Excerpt from Rick Rubin, Desert Island Discs, BBC Radio 4, 14 August 2022 © BBC; p. 81 Excerpt from Zadie Smith, 'Zadie Smith on Style', Vogue, 4 April 2024 © Condé Nast; p. 83 Quote from 'Shall we all be dopamine dressing?' by Amy de Klerk, Harper's Bazaar UK, 16 April 2021 © Hearst UK; p. 111 Excerpt from Michaela Coel's acceptance speech at the 73rd Primetime Emmy Awards, 19 September 2021; p. 115 Quotation from American Symphony, directed by Matthew Heineman © 2023 Netflix.

Edited by Jenni Davis
Designed and typeset by Vaidehi Tikekar
Cover design by Anna Morrison
Project management by Whitefox Publishing Limited

To my small circle of people who loved me through my year of nothing – without trying to fix or change me. Thank you.

CONTENTS

Foreword by Julia Cameron   13

Updated Author's Note, 2025   17

Author's Note, 2023   21

Winter | Spring

November   27
December   33
January   39
February   45
March   53
April   60
May   64

Summer | Autumn

June   71
July   78
August   84
September   93
October   99

Winter

November   107
December   113

Afterword   119

Acknowledgements   125

Foreword by Julia Cameron

For thirty-plus years, I have been writing Morning Pages: three daily pages of longhand writing about anything and everything. They have traced the track of my life. They have recorded ups and downs, periods of flow and times of apparent drought. They have given me a portal to a spiritual life, and they have led me to connect with kindred spirits – among them, Emma Gannon.

Gannon is a brave author, tackling subjects lesser writers prefer to ignore. Take the book you hold in your hands: *A Year of Nothing*. It details Gannon's nervous breakdown – a collapse that came to her at the zenith of her career. This confession opens Gannon's narrative. Suffering from panic attacks and a mysterious leaching of her normally high-powered energies, she marks a date: 22 October 2022.

She was plunged into a harrowing period of inertia. She writes, 'Even though we know deep down these periods of life are temporary, it is terrifying not knowing when it will end.' Her best friend tells her she looks 'frail', but she ignores the warning, papering over the cracks with a bold coat and red lipstick. The warning signs of an impending collapse met with Gannon's denial. After all, she had just handed in a new non-fiction book, *The Success Myth*. Ironically, it argued that 'success only feels good when it's also aligned with your heart'. Gannon's own success ignored the pleading of her heart for a slower, saner life. The collapse came, and Gannon found herself grappling with an existential breakdown. She took to her bed.

No longer 'busy, busy, busy', she was forced to look at the small things she had, in her busy-ness, overlooked: the green leaves of her houseplants, the smell of incense, the softness of a comforting blanket. A writer by temperament and habit, Gannon kept a diary throughout her year of nothing. She recorded her impressions of nothingness, taking care to note the drama of a life without moorings. Her descriptions of her own psyche were often frightening.

Moving through her altered life a month at a time, helped by her diary to recall specifics, Gannon wrote of what the poet Robert Bly called 'the descent into the ashes'.

A writer less bold than Gannon wouldn't trust readers to go along on her journey. Even Gannon herself found her trip harrowing. She admitted that she could sympathise with the impulse to avoid pain. An increased willingness to feel her feelings characterised Gannon's slow recovery. Inviting her readers to do the same, she doesn't mince words. She became addicted to cold water swimming, taking readers with her as she plunged into icy waters. Moving around the calendar year since her meltdown, Gannon recorded an increased hunger for clarity and decided to give up booze. One more time, trusting her readership to go along with her. Again, her candour smacks of bravery.

Foreword

Telling the story of her nervous breakdown from the inside out, Emma Gannon sets a heroic example. Her honesty, open-mindedness and willingness to be vulnerable lays out a path for her readers to follow.

Julia Cameron,
author of *The Artist's Way*, 2024

Updated Author's Note, 2025

I'm sitting here writing this from my kitchen table in London. The bamboo plants outside have grown a lot taller recently, and I have a bunch of flowers next to me, a gift from my agent, having just released a brand-new novel. I feel completely renewed – new hair, new perspective, and a settled nervous system. The trees on my street are full and green, with soft pink and white blossoms blooming right outside my window. I don't reference my year of nothing very often anymore, but for a couple of years it was all I could talk about, because my life had become so small and focused on recovery.

When I would bring it up at social events ('Sorry I've been AWOL, I couldn't work or do anything for months!'), I found many people would say to me: 'I'm so sorry, that sounds awful.' As much as that is a thoughtful response, it didn't feel quite right: because, yes, it was awful, and it was also *brilliant*. You only realise in hindsight that your breakdown was a breakthrough.

I find myself returning to something novelist Taffy Brodesser-Akner once said about the iconic screaming scene in *Fleishman Is in Trouble*, brought to life so excellently by Claire Danes in the TV adaptation:

'I'm a big fan of the nervous breakdown as a completely rational response,' Taffy said.

A nervous breakdown is a completely rational response! Yes. That landed in my body as truth. Life for many of us, and for very different personal reasons, is a lot. When I look back on this fallow year, recorded in the pages of this book, I do feel a sadness for the time that seemed 'lost' – but I also feel a deep and unexpected fondness.

It was a topsy-turvy, bedridden year of being adrift and wandering aimlessly, but I can't help but be grateful for it. Hard-won wisdom. Knowing that life goes on. That we have many micro and macro deaths of self within one lifetime. I'm no longer embarrassed about 'being too sensitive'.

A friend of mine, who had her burnout breakdown two years before I did, told me that one day I would feel like it's the best thing that ever happened to me. At the time, I couldn't believe that at all. And yet I had witnessed her own miracle unfold. A glorious transformation. I saw her in the park during her own 'year of nothing', make-up free, wearing an oversized cream fleece, walking her dog, looking empty, like a picture that needed colouring in. Big, impressive London job no more. No more clients. One day, she sent me a picture of her sitting at her window, letting the light in; she had herself some sunflowers, placed them in large vase, and had a paint set and a copy of *The Artist's Way*. She was finding a way to heal. I see her now, years on, living her life in a sunny European city, seeing now how her burnout re-routed her in a beautiful, dramatic way. Fewer spikes, more soft edges. She recently posted something online

Updated Author's Note, 2025

that said: *I'm the softest and most ruthless I've ever been.* That's how I feel. So much softer, and yet so much more powerful. Softening your edges doesn't mean you lose your spark; it eventually comes back to you.

I have so much to thank my year of nothing for. It taught me how to rest, how to heal, how to prioritise my health and how to trust myself. How to let go and see if a net might catch me. It taught me how to live. Learning how to live through such darkness, confusion and dissociation made me realise that if all my success and career went away tomorrow, I'd be OK, because I know now how to do the basics of life. It taught me how to prioritise, how to get down on the floor and surrender, and yet how to properly stand up for myself. It taught me who my friends are.

For so long I had compartmentalised my life, fracturing myself into different versions depending on the person I was with or the environment I was in. I would split myself down the middle between Work Self and Home Self, never introducing one to the other. When I came out the other side of this, I realised I'd combined all my different selves. They joined forces, they finally pulled up a pew and dined together, they had become friends. For the first time, I felt whole. One joined-together person. Recognised myself in the mirror again. What a relief. It was exhausting to keep so many plates spinning – to be so many versions of myself at once.

My friend Donna Lancaster always says: 'I trust completely in life.' This was new to me – the idea of trusting life, embracing the path, the natural ebb and flow, and having faith where it will lead you. My burnout episode re-routed me – now I join Donna in saying *I trust in life*. I know now that everything that happened was on my side. This 're-route' has sent me in the most magical direction.

This book, *A Year of Nothing*, is in many ways a love letter to my inner circle. My parents, my husband, my siblings, my best friends. It's also a gift for you. It was this year of nothingness that brought me right back to everything that is most important to me. I hope you enjoy this book; I'm so glad I wrote it, because I couldn't write it now that I'm better. Much of it now feels like a distant dream. This is why I write, to capture these chapters of life. Because often life feels like a butterfly constantly fluttering away, hard to grasp, impossible to pin down. Sometimes, though, it stays still long enough to have a proper magical glimpse up close.

This book will always be close to my heart, and writing it got me through a really crappy time in my life. Thank you for reading. Onwards.

Emma Gannon
June 2025

Author's Note, 2023

The Wanstead Flats stretched out before me – the grass once green was now parched and brown; crows circled overhead against a backdrop of wispy, lifeless clouds. A black dog ran free, the owner calling out their name. I was circling these open playing fields because I had nothing else to do. I focused on the birds in a nearby tree next to a pond, remembering that birdsong has historically always been a signal of safety for humans; it's meant to calm our nervous systems. No danger here. And yet, I did not feel safe.

This was one of many 'mental health' walks I took in 2023. I wore an oversized coat and scuffed-up Dr. Martens. During another mindless lap, I exchanged some WhatsApp voice notes back and forth with my friend JP Watson, the founder and editor of the Pound Project. We were keeping in touch; he'd just had a baby and I was taking a forced break from work, signed off with severe medically diagnosed burnout (of which

I'll explain more in this book). I had no choice but to stop everything and batten down the hatches. I said no to new opportunities, quit the successful podcast I'd hosted for six years, took a break from my management team and agents who ran my schedule, shrank my friendship group, put an out-of-office on, and quit everything for a bit, used my savings, put my phone on airplane mode. I couldn't look at a screen for longer than thirty seconds, my brain just didn't feel the same. It was as if a circuit somewhere inside was shutting down and rewiring itself.

Back in 2018, I published a book called *Sabotage* with the Pound Project and I enjoyed the experience immensely. It was a book all about my personal relationship with self-sabotage. The corporate publishing world can feel intimidating and intense at times, huge buildings and boardrooms and spreadsheets and deadlines and pressure. The freedom as a writer to publish a smaller book without constrictions felt like a dream. To my absolute gratitude and delight, thousands of people supported *Sabotage* and it was received well. In 2020, *Sabotage* was then acquired and republished with added material by the publisher Hodder & Stoughton and continues to sell well.

As I write this, I've just returned home from a book event in Lisbon, speaking at independent bookstore Salted Books, and I glimpsed *Sabotage* on the shelves, with its spotted green cover. It boosted my faith in small independent publishing and it's exciting that stories travel across different countries even if they aren't so-called 'big hitters'. Something that was simply born out of fun, creativity and love continues to find its people. As a writer and creative person, it felt important not to lose track of this magic. I cannot afford to lose the magic; some days I wonder if it's all I have in order to keep creating. These days, I'm finding this spark daily – speaking to my readers via my Substack newsletter 'The Hyphen', a platform in which they pay me directly for my writing. Writing my book *The Success Myth* was a reminder to myself that success only feels good when it's also aligned with the compass of my heart. True north.

JP and I had a call halfway through my burnout year. He asked if I wanted to do another project together and we bounced around some ideas and came up with a good one (I think we wanted to originally call it 'Quitter'). I so wanted to do another book with him. However, even though my heart was saying yes, my body was saying a firm no. After the call ended, I knew I didn't have the energy or strength to take it on. I felt depleted and deflated, angry and upset that I had no energy to work on writing projects that once lit me up. It clearly wasn't the right time; I was not well enough yet. I told JP I couldn't do it, then took myself back to bed. It worried me, this intense lack of capacity and broken feeling in my brain. A few months on, JP also confided in me that he was worried when he saw me on Zoom. 'You . . . didn't look like yourself,' he said. For any creative person who expresses themselves through words to survive, it felt maddening to not have the energy to read or write. Then, I decided to lean into it. So instead, I put my pen down. I cleared my schedule. I dipped into my savings, I slept, I borrowed friends' dogs, I ate bananas in bed, I bought miniature plants, I read magazines. I lay down. For the first time in my entire life, I did nothing.

This book isn't the original idea JP and I had discussed, but instead, something more stripped back and truthful has been born.

This is *A Year of Nothing*.

Emma Gannon
October 2023

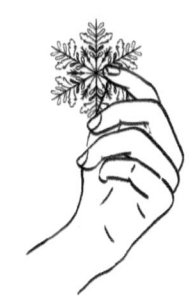

Winter

November

TO-DO LIST:

Lie in bed
Watch Sister Act *and* Sister Act 2

My burnout episode started unexpectedly during a relaxing spa weekend with a close friend at a hotel in the heart of the New Forest. She'd just got married and had recently hosted a mehndi at her house. We danced and had henna painted onto our hands. In celebratory mode, we'd booked ourselves into a gorgeous room with a four-poster bed and had just had a massage. During the massage I felt strange, different; the hands that touched my shoulders felt disembodied, floating. After the massage there was a miniature pool, overlooking the forest trees, with herbal remedies in the water, soaking into our skin. I was floating, drifting. Something didn't feel quite right.

A few nights before, I'd gone out for dinner in London Bridge with this same friend. When I walked in, she said: 'You OK? You look frail.' Frail. Fragile. A shell. She'd not used that word before to describe me.

I had my favourite coat on, red with a leopard-print trim, with matching red lipstick. Put a glossy Band-Aid over it. What could she see? I had just handed in a new book. *Busy, busy, busy. How are you? / Yeah, I'm fine! Bit overwhelmed, but hey, that's life! Everyone's busy.*

Although the years of the Covid-19 lockdowns were unpredictable and scary, they also suited my introverted nature much better. I liked having a smaller life. I found relief in having so many cancellations. But then the world was back open and so – like many others – I felt I needed to 'make up for lost time'. There was a collective vibe of *pack the diary full.*

Dinner reservations. Get married. Book promo ideas. Plans for 2023. Colour-coded diary. Write another novel. Sign contract. Weekends away. DMs from strangers. Requests. Friends' weddings. Mortgage rates. Let's have a brainstorm. Should do some exercise. Have I left the hob on? Emails. Friend's birthday. Urgent response needed. Invoices. Life coach training! Dentist. Read the news. Don't read the news. Off to see family. Book flight to a book festival. Zoom call. Dinner in Soho. New work request. Rescue remedy. Take your vitamins. Let's get an Uber! More emails. Do you want to come on Good Morning Britain? *Tax return. Friend's birthday. Cost-of-living crisis. Builders in the house. Life. Life. Life.*

Does reading that paragraph make you feel anxious? Of course it does. And it's obvious why. So many of us are full to the brim. When was the last time I stretched my body or went for a walk? It all felt like such a lot suddenly (and unlike many of my friends, I don't even have kids.) I am financially stable. I work for myself. I am fortunate. *I shouldn't complain,* the voice said. So, onwards I went, not knowing how to stop, like a little mule up a steep mountain with so much luggage on my back, and every night I'd go to bed and think about my diary while my stomach did backflips and my thoughts were whizzing around my brain like a Scalextric.

Back to the New Forest. I was with my close friend C. I have known her since we were four years old and our families are friends. After the massage I was drifting away mentally in the swimming pool and then later at dinner had the worst panic attack of my life. *How embarrassing and ungrateful*, the voice said, *having a mental breakdown at a luxury hotel*.

I excused myself for the bathroom, sat on the loo trying to focus on breathing in and out. After the frantic pacing, still with difficulty breathing and clammy hands, I sat back down at dinner. C looked worried. I told her to stop looking worried. Then the waiter came over and he looked blurry in my vision and started fading away too. He was pixelated, a floating head without a body. I needed to go back to the room and lie down.

According to all those therapy Instagram accounts, you're not meant to look worried when someone is having a panic attack, you're meant to gently remind them to breathe. I don't blame C for looking concerned though. The colour had completely drained from my face, my eyes were wide like a frightened animal.

On the drive back to London from the hotel, C put on a Céline Dion album (one of our favourites since our teen years) and I tried to rest, tried not to spiral into more anxiety about what was wrong. We had planned to go to a neighbouring restaurant for lunch, which had its own farm and produce and even pigs, but I was desperate to get home. I felt bad cutting the trip short, but I was in true fight-or-flight mode. I did not want to be on the motorway and closed my eyes tight. I felt like I was zipping through space on an out-of-control rocket ship. We stopped off at a service station. We got some snacks and a Starbucks and I went to the bathroom, and on the back of the door were sketches and doodles – 'Lucy Woz 'Ere' and 'RIP Taz' and other scribbles – but in different coloured biro pen I saw a list of positive affirmations scribbled all over:

Put yourself first.

You are loved.

Your feelings are valid!

Be kind to yourself.

It's OK to say NO!

Having boundaries doesn't make you mean.

TALK TO SOMEONE.

I burst into tears. At a toilet door! I was delirious and exhausted. I thought this was the universe speaking to me through the medium of grubby graffiti. Angels from the past telling me it's going to be OK. Everything felt dream-like. I needed to get into bed. I needed to talk to someone.

When I got home, I lay in bed for a week. I didn't recognise myself in my camera phone and I took a selfie to document how dead I looked behind the eyes. (I still struggle to look back at those photos, how visible it is that my spark had diminished.) During this time, not knowing how ill I'd become, my husband had organised for our garden to be redone. He'd designed everything himself on Photoshop and found a team of garden designers to bring it to life. Builders charged through our house, in big boots, carrying large olive trees through the kitchen. New shrubs were planted into soil: jasmine, ferns, hebe, blueberry plants, alliums. Fresh water helped everything to grow. By contrast, I felt like I was fading away. I couldn't even offer the builders a cup of tea. *Who's that strange woman upstairs who never comes down?* is what I imagined them saying.

In Claudia Hammond's *The Art of Rest*, she explains that although seeing loved ones is nourishing and one of the greatest joys of life, for many of us it is not actually *rest*. In the research-based 'rest test' list of nourishing-based activities, it's actually quite far down the bottom. At the top of the list are things like walking, nature, reading, listening to music. Solitary acts. It makes sense then, why all my plans with friends and family were actually depleting me more and more, why I was falling asleep at friends' houses, why my trips away weren't replenishing me, why work events were making me feel jittery and sick. I was like an overheated iPhone on 1 per cent battery with my body sending such extreme signals. Wow, our bodies are so dramatic sometimes! Was there any need for these severe panic attacks? Could it be the only way my body could force me to stop? Maybe I'm lucky. Maybe my body was trying to save my life.

When I'd gathered the strength, I made phone calls. One to my agent cancelling absolutely everything; one to a close childhood friend telling her I couldn't come to her wedding that weekend (this was so out of character that everyone knew it must be serious); one to my mum/dad telling them I was unwell and one to a GP (who diagnosed me with anxiety and burnout within minutes). I said the same thing to all: *I know I look like everything is always fine all the time. But it's not.*

'We just assumed you were a superwoman,' one of my agents said to me afterwards. 'Until suddenly you weren't.' Had I dehumanised myself? I remember snapping at a fellow author months earlier too, who'd said to me, 'You're a machine!' She said it as a compliment. 'No, I'm not,' I replied bluntly, with a bitter taste in my mouth.

I went back to bed with a sinking feeling in my stomach but simultaneously a sense of huge relief. I turned off my phone. Social media and the constant noise evaporated into thin air. I needed a break from everyone else's lives to focus on my own. My phone slid under my bed. It felt like an odd relief, to be too ill to look at screens or type.

In Martha Beck's *The Way of Integrity*, she said that telling lies makes us ill. Not being our true selves comes at a cost. Pretending makes us ill. Work, productivity and achievement had become my coping mechanisms. Writhing and wriggling about in bed, it was like I was going through withdrawal. But it wasn't a habit of alcohol or drugs that I needed to kick, it was work and people-pleasing. These were my substances of choice, my numbing agent, and something that society also reinforces through praise and money. A friend in the industry said to me (which her therapist had said to her): 'What got you here won't get you there.' What worked well before will no longer work now. Things have to change. Boundaries were being formed. You are melting and rebuilding your life.

December

TO-DO LIST:

Stop everything
Watch Christmas films
Read Rest, Pause, Be
by Octavia F. Raheem

I've always found podcasts relaxing, the intimate nature of the host speaking directly to you. It's as though you are part of a conversation, but you don't have to talk. Kirsty Young, former host of *Desert Island Discs*, has a BBC Radio 4 podcast called *Young Again*, where she interviews celebrities on advice they'd give their younger selves. Actress Jada Pinkett Smith is one of the guests and she talks about her first proper breakdown in the 1990s. She explains there was no conversation happening about mental health back then, especially in the Black community. When Jada is asked what she'd tell her younger self, she says: 'I know you're having a hard time and I know this is unlike anything you've ever felt, but this is just your soul and your spirit telling you that there's a lot to look at.' I thought it was such a poetic and practical way of looking at it.

After suffering panic attacks at night for a while, I felt like I was looking at a stranger and it freaked me out. Was it my spirit asking me to take a look at things? I had read before about dissociative symptoms and they are usually linked to post-traumatic stress disorder, even though I didn't feel like I had anything to have PTSD about. My therapist later explained how we can have a build-up of micro-traumas over time. Another therapist explained the phrase 'window of tolerance' to me (your specific zone in which you can handle stress calmly). We all have different acceptance levels of what life throws at us, regardless of the specifics. Some people can have three hours of sleep at night and a stressful job and just not get tired, some people can get exhausted by twenty minutes of small talk. Social media is faster and crazier than ever. We live in a world where we are fed 24/7 coverage of hideous news. No wonder we're feeling traumatised and terrified.

Dissociation is horrible. You live in an upside-down world where nothing really makes sense. Everything looked like a cardboard cutout. A spooky Disneyland. Alien and two-dimensional. I'd look out of a train window and convince myself it was a digital screen. I'd find myself knocking on a wooden table, trying to convince myself it was real. I felt like a floating particle that didn't have a home inside my own body. Where had I gone? When we say, 'I don't really feel like myself at the moment,' what do we really mean by this? What and who is 'myself'? And where is she?

Dissociation feels like disconnection from everything and everyone, including the planet and the universe and yourself: like you are watching a film and losing your grasp on reality.

In short, you don't believe in anything anymore.

✻✻✻

Thank goodness for December. A respite, a breather, a year end; the Christmas lights are up, the out-of-office is on. On paper, it is a great time to do nothing. In reality, it's usually a time of more stress, more admin, more to-do lists. But for Christmas 2022, I decided to opt out. I could not make the effort, it was impossible. My nervous system felt mangled and when I lifted my arms, my fingers tingled, the nerves not quite reaching as far as they once did. My limbs were stiff. When I uncurled my fingers from a fist, my fingers would feel rigid and electric. I got pins and needles constantly. My body wasn't working smoothly or effortlessly like before; everything felt fraught, as though it was trying to rebuild or rewire itself. I kept googling my symptoms and reading that famous line: *It's probably nothing – but it may be a sign of a more serious underlying health condition.*

I have always felt alienated from yoga culture – I would walk past the Lululemon women in my neighbourhood, with their swinging sleek ponytails and smoothies and designer yoga mats, and feel like we were a different species. The tight, freshly washed leggings and early mornings and headstands, how?

During this frazzled time, when my body felt disconnected from my brain, my body took over. It looked after me. It was on autopilot. It would get me out of bed, walk me into my study, light a candle, get a mat out, type in 'gentle yoga'. I found a woman who did cosy yoga in a massive grey hoodie and joggers and used pillows and blankets as part of the stretching, with her dog lying next to her. No designer leggings in sight. Soft and gentle movement. I needed a judgement-free zone. I was swaddling myself back to health.

I felt lucky I could retreat into my family cocoon over Christmas. My husband did all the heavy lifting with Mum, Dad, sister and brother-in-law coming over. He cooked two massive turkey crowns (one on Christmas Day for my family, and one on Boxing Day for his family). I did nothing. I shrivelled up into my festive jumper and everyone accepted I was going through something – even though the something felt strange and invisible – and was incredibly understanding. I quietly ate potatoes in the corner. I found the fairy lights on the Christmas tree relaxing. With most invisible illnesses, you don't look different; you might have greasy hair and a puffy face, but you can talk and breathe and eat and walk. But I knew in my bones that something big was shifting inside. Something I couldn't really explain. I started to get tinnitus.

It snowed during this December and thick inches created a white blanket on everything in the garden. It started snowing late into the night, and at midnight, instead of going to bed, my husband and I wrapped ourselves up in our big coats and went outside and just marvelled at it. The snowflakes fell onto my cheeks and onto my tongue and in that moment I felt like things were going to be OK, but only if I could engage with the realities of the world properly and honestly. Only if I really saw the world around me, really saw nature and people and the elements and felt the hot and the cold and the good and the bad. No more shying away from everything. I touched the leaves on a newly sprouting plant that made its way through the snow and felt a small ripple of hope. The assignment was clear: the world was dark at times, but it was also extremely magical, and it was possible to hold both together in one palm.

❄ ❄ ❄

A couple of years before, in 2021, I'd taken my mum to New York to see the Christmas lights and the dazzling displays along Fifth Avenue. I had tickets to see Candace Bushnell's one-woman show at a Union Square theatre and asked Mum if she wanted to come with me. We'd both enjoyed *Sex and the*

City and my mum always enjoys a sparkly outfit and a cocktail. The pandemic was still happening, but we could go if we were vaccinated and wore masks everywhere. My energy levels were low, and I found myself needing to go back to my room for naps, a lot. Mum commented on my energy levels; I wondered if I needed a blood test. I wondered if my burnout symptoms had been creeping up for years. I started to notice this increasingly urgent desire to be alone. My agent emailed me some good news: I'd just had a book proposal accepted for *The Success Myth*, a non-fiction title unpicking all the lies we'd been told about what makes us happy in modern work culture. When I thought about the commitments I'd made to my publisher to promote the book, I just wanted to fall asleep right away.

My mum loves Christmas. Specifically, Christmas films and hunting for a new shiny Christmas decoration. Every year, without fail, we watch *Miracle on 34th Street*. The 1994 version with Mara Wilson as the little girl and Richard Attenborough as Santa aka Kris Kringle. 'Cole's' is the fictional department store in the film, based on Macy's. It is a film about the concept of Santa and whether or not he is 'real'. In the courtroom, Mara Wilson and her lawyer stepfather (well, future stepfather) are trying to prove Santa is real using 'evidence'. This 'proving' of Santa is like trying to suggest evidence for God. The question is: do we need proof in order to believe?

A huge part of human life is the embracing of the mystery of it all and the incessant need to find answers. There is an 'unknown' at play. The idea of believing in Santa as a child is like wanting to believe in something bigger than yourself once you're an adult. Believing feels good. As Einstein reportedly once said: 'The most important decision we make is whether we believe we live in a friendly or a hostile universe.'

After eating copious amounts of chocolate with tea and drinking big tumblers of Baileys on Christmas Eve, we all went up to bed. Mum texted me from the spare bedroom, right at the top of my house:

'Remember when we saw this, last year?'

She attached a picture of the outside of Macy's with 'BELIEVE' written in huge lit-up letters on the side of the store. It felt like a sign. (A literal sign.) *Believe*.

Believe. I was starting to realise that no matter what you believed – whether you think you're awful or brilliant – the reality (people, physics, buildings, weather, materials) around you stays the same. Essentially, you are what you believe. As my friend Leyla says, 'Whether you think you can, or you think you can't – you're right.' I wasn't able to implement it yet, or do away with my bad thoughts, but the seed was being sown.

As Ann Patchett writes in her memoir *Truth and Beauty*: 'It takes a lot of energy to be miserable and a lot of energy to be sad, which one are you going to choose?'

OVER TO YOU

Who/what do you believe in?

Do you believe in magic?

Do you ever make time to daydream and wonder?

Do you believe in yourself?

January

TO-DO LIST:

Watch Save the Last Dance
*Look after Betty
(a miniature Dachshund)
Book a city break (and do
nothing once there)*

How did my New Year begin? From my bed, propped up by countless pillows like a grandparent from *Charlie and the Chocolate Factory*, I tried to look for clues. Those weeks leading up to my meltdown – how did I miss the warning signs? Earlier, in the summer of 2022, I had been away in California on a family holiday and while everyone else was having fun, wine tasting, karaoke, dancing by the pool, I felt my head pulsate like a balloon full of too much water. The karaoke microphones were too loud. I needed to go outside and take in gulps of air. My dad, tipsy and merry, grabbed my shoulder playfully and told me to lighten up. He didn't mean any harm, but I cried on the way home because that's what I desperately wanted: to lighten up.

The next day, I tried to distract myself by reading a hardcore self-help book on the beach and my headache and dissociation got worse. Why didn't I just put the book down and look out at the sea? Why couldn't I relax? It's like my body had gone past the point of no return. I think my body was asking me to look around and take in the magical scenery instead of having my head in a textbook. *Look at me*, it was saying. *Look at the mountains, the sea, the sky.*

I had zero capacity for fun. I couldn't let myself off the hook. I was adamant on stuffing more and more information into my brain. It was like I was in fight-or-flight mode, trapped inside an endless scroll.

But how? How do you relax and have fun when you've fallen down a deep, dark well? The holiday was following a busy summer, home renovations, my wedding, and three of my best friends' weddings. My wedding had been reorganised many times due to the pandemic in 2021, and due to stress I had also failed to hand in a second novel on time. Everyone else was sunbathing and enjoying the fact that the world was back open again. I sat by the pool googling things such as:

What is reality?

Is your reality the only reality?

How does consciousness work?

Meaning of life?

Dark matter

Black holes

I wouldn't make a very good detective. I have looked on my camera roll for signs of my breakdown happening. I suppose, if I look very closely, I do look slightly dishevelled. Split ends. Bags under my eyes. Spaced-out pupils. Clashing clothes that weren't easy on the eye (cry for help?). I used an obscene amount of Lush bath bombs. Looking back now, I can see that I was unwell, and beyond the point of exhaustion. My eyelids were constantly aching, wanting to close. My body felt like a big, heavy lump.

A red flag: I didn't want to see my friends on New Year's Eve and I always want to see my friends on New Year's Eve. This was a warning sign. I see the same group of friends every year without fail, it's become a tradition. In our twenties, we used to dance around my small east-London flat, making 'dubsmash' videos to 'Hotline Bling', drinking too much and being ridiculous. And now in our thirties, we have dinner parties with good food, great wine, and beautifully set tables. Nowadays, small babies and toddlers who refuse to sleep join in the party too. We are growing older together, marked by the turn of the new year, so it felt truly odd not to be together. I spent the start of the year in bed, watching fireworks outside my window, completely alone. I told my husband to go still; I didn't want to ruin his fun. Go and have fun without me.

I hated the fireworks. I was angry at them. I felt like a scared dog, under the covers, thinking about the actual dogs who would also be hating them. Why is everything so noisy and loud? Why is everything suddenly making me jump? Why is everything so intense and in my face? How are other people happy and stress-free?

The other sign that something wasn't OK: people sent me gifts! I didn't have a broken leg, but they knew something bad was up. My friend Abbie sent me a beautiful candle, Kim sent me flowers and a note, Sian sent bath salts, my sister, Jo, sent me some chocolate, a colleague sent a small hamper of goodies, and a yellow candle from my friend C. 'Friends' who would only get in touch when I was 'doing well' drifted away.

On 5 January, I booked myself a flight via the British Airways sale. The brief was: I want to see something beautiful.

I booked a hotel room with a good view in Porto, a coastal city in Portugal known for its big bridges and port wine production. I wanted to start the new year by choosing myself. I felt wobbly and anxious still, but it felt like the right amount of pushing outside of my comfort zone.

Many people go on city breaks with a 'to-do' list from Condé Nast Traveller in their back pocket, a tick-list of sightseeing, but the point of this trip, for me, was to do nothing. My only plan was to arrive, check in to the hotel, sleep, eat and then walk each day. And watch the world go by. I only needed a few days. I knew it would help.

I stayed at what is apparently Porto's 'sexiest hotel': the Torel Avantgarde. I thought it would make me feel like I was a main character in my story again. It also won Best View at a recent small hotel awards, and I could see why – a sparkling pool below overlooked a lake dotted with boats, surrounded by orange-hued buildings and lemon trees. Every room was named after a creative pioneer. I stayed in the Oskar Barnack room, a photographer who built the first commercially successful camera in 1913. Golden sunlight flooded the bedroom each morning, inviting me to get up and seize the day. I took a dip in the pool and it was freezing, every cell in my body zinging to life. Breakfast was indulgent (pastel de nata, doughnuts, bagels, different types of doughy bread, tiers of chocolate cake) and it was walking distance from all the town action. I had to go up steep little hills and down lots of steps. My legs needed it after spending weeks in bed.

I visited the most beautiful bookstore in the world, Livraria Lello, also known as the cathedral of books, founded in 1869 by the French publisher and bookseller Ernesto Chardron. I got lost on the walk back to my hotel and walked straight into a botanical garden with vibrant colours, fountains, sculptures, magnolias, mosaics and big olive trees.

Winter

I walked for an hour along the waterfront, not knowing I would shortly end up at a little beach café. I was the only one there for hours. I headed to Restaurante Praia da Luz, a nondescript simple café overlooking a small beach. I sat in the town square alone with a coffee, listening to live modern jazz music (a saxophone player playing Dua Lipa covers), got on the tram for fun, didn't drink alcohol, took Liz Gilbert's new-year workshop late one night in my hotel room, and listened to *Desert Island Discs* on repeat. I know I didn't scratch the surface of what beautiful Porto has to offer because I just walked aimlessly around – but I didn't care. I didn't want a to-do list; the views alone filled me up. I wanted to just be.

Walking on the beach, a song came on to my Spotify shuffle that I've always found sad. 'This Bitter Earth/On the Nature of Daylight', a song by Dinah Washington and Max Richter. It's one of those songs that gets to the crux of the great symphony of life, and I often can't listen to it in full, I have to turn it off. My husband loves the song and tried to explain that it's about how Earth can seem bitter and dark at first glance, but in reality, it also bears so much glorious fruit – showing how both can be true at the same time. He believes it is a hopeful song. Looking out at the ocean, the wind messing up my hair, the sea air making my eyes stream, I pressed play and played it in full. I leant all the way in. I felt all my feelings for the first time in ages. I didn't shy away. I let it completely take over. I let all the emotions wash over me. It felt painful but it felt cathartic. I realised in that precise moment that I had entered into a new portal. I was beginning to lean more deeply into life. No more blocking out reality, and all the different rainbow colours and feelings it brings. A friend of mine said that when you are peeling off a new layer you might feel some turbulence, because you are shifting up a gear.

OVER TO YOU

*What does 'doing nothing' on a trip
away look like to you?*

Would you book a solo trip for a couple of nights?

*What playlists do you have to suit
your different moods?*

February

TO-DO LIST:

Walk around graveyards
Be sad

We shouldn't need to go away somewhere in order to do nothing, but sometimes it can help. It enables us to shut the door on our life for a bit. It is romanticised too, sold to us all the time. Big posters on the Tube of blue skies, white sand and turquoise water; discounted trips via Ryanair. Holidays, staycations, hotels, resorts, retreats that promise us the headspace to be totally alone and calm and peaceful. Treehouses, in particular, always lure me in. The idea of a wooden Wendy house in the sky, surrounded by birds, with cows and sheep in the surrounding fields, away from everything, in a small town in the UK called Tickle Cock Bridge or a place that doesn't sound real. Images on Instagram with influencers in bed with their Stanley cups, someone reading a book by a log fire with beautiful greenery out of a big square window. Link in bio. Sold. Expensive. Ouch. This is how bad we are at the concept of 'doing nothing': it has to be packaged up and sold. Surely switching off can be done anywhere? Surely we don't need to spend money all the time, in order to do nothing?

I remember, when I was ten, my mum and dad asking me and my sister to come into the kitchen. They had a surprise for us and were looking sheepish, standing in the middle of the room, nudging each other, smiling. We were then taken down to the bottom of the garden, and they wouldn't give us a clue. What could it be? A new pet? We passed my mum's tomato-filled greenhouse and went down some steps, and there it was (my mouth hung open with shock): a small wooden treehouse above our heads. Dad had asked his builder friend (genuinely called Bob) to assemble one for us. My heart skipped a beat.

It was perfect. It had a tiny little green rope ladder going up, swinging in the breeze, and a small entrance via a square wooden carved-out hole. The little house itself was just big enough for my sister and me to sit in, with our knees to our chest, chatting. We brought pillows and blankets and teddies with us. It was the most exciting thing. A hideaway to do nothing. I think this is why treehouses can have such a nostalgic pull when we're adults. For me, and I feel so lucky, it was my first hiding place.

❋ ❋ ❋

During this month of February, three old school friends and I arrived at a treehouse in Glastonbury, Somerset. Two of my friends' birthdays are in February so it's normally a good month for us to go away together. It's something we've done regularly over the past five years. We've stayed in treehouses, huts, even an old traveller's wagon, and the idea is getting back to nature, making simple breakfasts together, doing face masks, reading magazines in bed, eating in pubs, going cold swimming in a nearby lake, getting out of London for a few days and just being together. We booked a 'back to basics' treehouse this time – an outdoor shower, no working kitchen, a wood-fire bath, a chess set, a log burner, a kettle that takes hours to heat up, that kind of thing. When we arrived, it was pitch black. We'd parked in a big open field and had to make our way down to the treehouse in the dark with only our phone torches for assistance. My friend's car got stuck in the mud and so we abandoned it in the field; we'd worry about it later. It felt symbolic – we were venturing into the darkness. Physically and emotionally.

It didn't take long to realise that all four of us were feeling miserable and disconnected. We were happy to be together on the surface, but no one had the energy to really make much of an effort. We went for food at a local pub and ordered burgers. One friend was distracted, freshly out of a long relationship, chatting to someone on a dating app. Another friend was texting her husband under the table. The other was staring into space, then replying to work emails with a fast-moving thumb. I went outside for some air, anxiety building in my chest. Our weekend of fun wasn't looking so fun.

It's calming and confronting, spending time with friends you've known since you were very young. And yet I felt distant and separate from them in that moment. Were we clinging on to the past?

I look at these old friends and notice more laughter lines and wrinkles around our eyes. We've all been through more stuff now. We are no longer 'young'. Our worlds are now full of either fertility conversations, existential thoughts, health scares or kids. We've all changed. I notice there are certain things about each other that we no longer understand. I notice that life suddenly got hard. We no longer have carefree nights out to gossip or tell private jokes about boys at school, or share common-room nonchalance. No more obvious commonalities. Our lives got more serious, but the love is still there. But at this point in our lives, we are struggling to be there for each other. Each of us has our own particular brand of discomfort and stress and there is no clear ringleader.

We sat around the wooden table in the treehouse trying so hard to make light conversation, stoking the fire, pouring drinks, playing cards, but it kept coming back to mental health, job stress, unhappiness. It wasn't easy to connect, and things didn't flow. There wasn't much laughter, and we usually laugh a lot together. We spent the weekend lying around while it rained, mostly on our phones in bed, sharing memes, each trying to steady ourselves. *This is it*, I thought to myself, *this is the beginning of getting older; of shit getting real*. We used to have it so easy.

When I got home to my husband, I realised that I didn't have a good time and at first I felt guilty about this. I was so relieved not to be at the treehouse anymore. Of course, the photos on my phone told a different story; I'd managed to take some pictures of us smiling next to the outdoor bath and posted them on Instagram. It was no reflection of my friends, but I just wanted to be alone. I felt more ringing in my ears – and when I googled it, I got two answers. A medical site said it could be to do with 'a build-up of earwax', and an answer from a spiritual blog said it was because I was having a 'deep awakening'.

Maybe I was trying to force people together like the 'good old times', and I had yet to accept that they no longer existed. Or at least, had changed. Time to step away, slow down. This wasn't a friendship break-up situation, but maybe a friendship 'break'. Maybe it was time also to widen my network, invite new friends in.

✽ ✽ ✽

Things were falling away. After the treehouse experience, I spent more time alone. I visited graveyards a lot during this month. I would just end up there on a walk, as if my body was following an invisible compass: St Patrick's Roman Catholic Cemetery, Leytonstone, where apparently Alfred Hitchcock is buried. I remember walking around the stone path, feeling guided, almost like I was being given a tour of the graves, taking in all the different names, birth dates and ages of the deceased. Respect the dead, respect death. It felt like a force carried me around in a circle, making me look and pay attention. Graveyards are normally associated with horror films or green monsters or Halloween, but there was nothing scary about it at all. It felt extremely peaceful. It was a beautiful day, with sunlight filtering through the trees and shining gently on the graves. I was mourning myself, my old life, my old self, my past. Things were dying off, and I was making space for what was to come next.

OVER TO YOU

Make a list of friends/people who you feel totally comfortable with, who you could invite round to have a 'doing nothing' day together.

What do you need to mourn, or let go of?

Who, and what, is no longer serving you?

Spring

March

TO-DO LIST:

Book a reflexology session

On a bad day, I rang the NHS, but the GP didn't really have time to get into my issues properly. I had a quick five-minute phone call and without asking me any questions she offered me anti-anxiety medication. (I am all for people taking medication when they need it, I celebrate and encourage this – but for me, it didn't feel right. It felt like it should be a last resort; I hadn't tried enough other avenues yet). Five minutes surely wasn't enough time to reach a conclusion. There were no holistic questions, no context, no understanding, no wider reflections. No questions about job, diet, movement, life, mental health symptoms, I wanted to try getting back to the basics first. I felt palmed off, dismissed and frustrated. Instead, they sent me a series of texts afterwards from my GP's practice:

> Dear Emma,
> Are you still feeling stressed and overwhelmed? Keep an eye out on our website for some friendly tips!

They were overrun and short-staffed and trying their best. My frustration wasn't on the individuals who worked there, it was on the system at large. I rang BUPA and paid £80 for an hour's consultation with a doctor instead. They were helpful this time, as you'd expect with an expensive pay-as-you-go rate. I was diagnosed with anxiety and burnout. She took me through the Generalised Anxiety Test (I scored high) and told me I needed time off work and that my nervous system needed time to repair. No pills pushed onto me (and I want to acknowledge again that I know this can work wonders for other people in different situations); I wanted a better understanding of the anxiety moving around my body and how to navigate it better. Even though she diagnosed me with GAD, I knew deep down that my anxiety was temporary and circumstantial. I didn't want to stick a label-for-life onto myself. Human beings go through changes and transitions and it is terrifying, but I knew I had to ride it out. I felt relieved to have spoken to a kind medical professional who listened and gave me time to talk, but also disappointed, knowing that there are people who wouldn't be able to afford the private fee.

I continued doing all the right things: lying on the sofa, looking after a dog, going swimming, watching the Disney channel, but I wasn't feeling any better. My husband was amazing, offering kindness and patience and not trying to 'fix' me, but he couldn't just lie around with me, he had his own work and life to be getting on with. I asked him recently if he was worried about me at the time, the fact that I couldn't function for months. He said it felt instinctively like something I was 'going through'. I found this so refreshing, this idea that I didn't need to 'hurry up' and get better. It definitely helped: the fact that he knew I'd be OK eventually. But I was frustrated at how 'long' my recovery was taking. A friend of mine said that

Spring

severe burnout usually takes a year minimum to recover from, and I didn't believe her at the time.

One afternoon, I found myself walking down the road adjacent to my house and stumbling across a tiny little spa. I must have walked past it a million times but never really noticed it before. It was nondescript, except for a purple sign and a few 'Voted Best Spa 2019' signs in the window. I booked in for a reflexology session with a woman named Isabel.

I'm a huge fan of alternative therapies. In 2022, I signed up to take Martha Beck's life-coaching course. Life coaching has a notoriously bad rap, with so many charlatans and uncertified courses floating about, but Beck is the real deal – with three degrees from Harvard, and having been Oprah Winfrey's coach, she is someone who really walks the walk. During the nine-month course, I met a group of women who were incredibly supportive and lots of different kinds of therapeutic practitioners. Several women from my course supported me in ways I hadn't expected – one offered Reiki over Zoom, another was a thoughtful and grounded grief counsellor, and another brought deep insight through her Enneagram work. I felt myself becoming increasingly connected to these intuitive, kind, empathetic friends. One of them always ended our calls with the words: *'You're right where you need to be.'* They all checked in on me. Our WhatsApp group became a bit of a life raft.

I thought back to the practitioners who helped me in previous life hurdles. The man who did my acupuncture when I kept getting UTIs. A kind Tarot reader I met on a retreat. The incredible reflexologist named Cee near my old house in Hackney, who could foresee when I would have my period, or get a cold, always predicting correctly to the exact day. After massaging my feet and somehow looking into my soul, she would need to leave the room for a minute and have a sit-down. She was very intuitive. She once told me she detected her friend's early cancer during a session and didn't know how to tell her. Sadly, she'd left the practice, moved back to Spain and her WhatsApp number no longer worked.

Reflexology felt more spiritual than a massage, with its focus on the connection of the foot to the rest of the body. Although the practice is yet to have major scientific backing, it's said that massaging the big toe is connected to your brain, the bottom of your foot to your pelvic area, the area just underneath your toes with the chest. According to traditional Chinese medicine, these points are believed to reduce stress, help digestion and promote good sleep hygiene.

Finding Isabel, a reflexologist in my local neighbourhood, felt magical and timely. A petite Turkish woman with reddish spiky hair, I liked her immediately and she asked me to lie down on the bed. When I started choking up, crying, tears streaming down my face and into my ears, I felt embarrassed. I wanted to keep a lid on it, but I couldn't. Everything was bubbling over, and maybe she was bringing it out of me through her kind, understanding presence. Isabel clearly wasn't interested in pretences. In that room, I could be exactly who I was in that moment. She didn't panic or ask me any questions, she just placed her hands on me.

I felt a deep shame about my state, the ugly crying, the spots on my chin, the broken hair around my ears, my involuntary vulnerability and how exposing it seemed, breaking down in front of a stranger.

She stepped around to the back of the table and stroked my hair in silence.

'You have too many thoughts,' she said neutrally.

Spring

At the time, this felt unhelpful. I couldn't think straight. I couldn't just get rid of my thoughts. She carried on stroking my hair.

'The universe has it covered.' She said it with such belief. 'You will be OK.'

She massaged my legs and pushed deeply into the soles of my feet, but I was unable to switch off. Usually, during my previous sessions with Cee, I could totally drift off into a deep trance and state of relaxation. But this time, I was too tetchy; I felt so uncomfortable inside my body.

I cried at the end, because I felt so moved by this stranger using her skills to relax me. How she had massaged my feet, then my hands, then my head. 'I don't know what's wrong with me. I'm normally quite positive,' I spluttered through throaty tears. This was the problem. *I'm normally quite positive.* I was in a shame spiral. I had swallowed that message from childhood whole: that if I wasn't positive, happy and productive then I wasn't of value.

'Come back and see me in a month,' Isabel said, and she handed me a small bottle of frankincense. When I looked up what frankincense is used for, it said 'relieves chronic stress and anxiety'.

I wrote 'the universe has it covered' on a piece of paper and kept it by my bed that night. I felt embarrassed at how much I was hanging on to the words of this woman, who I'd only just met.

During this time, I also went to see a woman who did craniosacral therapy in my local area. I didn't know what to expect, except that it involved 'gentle touch'. I went to her little studio, a ten-minute walk from my house, and she took off her shoes and cupped my body in places, closing her eyes, holding her hands on me in areas of my body. She placed her hands very slowly under my lower back, the idea being that it would alleviate tension. I closed my eyes and felt my body contort to one side, but when I opened my eyes, I was still lying straight.

Afterwards, I felt so much better. Was my energy moving around the room? Did she actually do anything – or was it lying on a bed with someone gently placing her hands on me? Was it just the act of lying down and being held by a kind stranger? Did it matter?

A few weeks later, I visited Isabel again. She didn't say much, just nodded and told me I was slowly getting better. She told me I'd gained weight, but she was smiling, pleased. Stress had eaten away at me and made my face gaunt, she said. Much better now. 'Your baby hairs are growing back slowly.' She'd noticed that my hair had become thin around my ears, another sign of chronic stress.

She told me that during the first session she was worried, that I was at a crossroads, and was heading towards depression.

'Everything was so dark for you,' she said.

But then, she could see that I managed to turn a corner. She was beaming at me, telling me I was getting better now and wouldn't feel like that again. I chose to believe her. I couldn't unlearn what I'd learnt about burnout and recovery. This new information was helpful, I was grateful for it.

Record producer Rick Rubin speaks about his own breakdown, when he was thirty-three, the same age as I was, on BBC Radio 4's *Desert Island Discs*. I listened to it on my earlier trip to Porto, while waiting for a delayed flight home. He said:

> *I went through a depression for the first time in my life; it wasn't anything that I understood, I thought I was dying. I was going to see a therapeutic practitioner of one kind or another, probably two to five days a week. I would drag myself out of bed, in the hope this was going to fix it, and that was my life for two years.*

There was this primal need to fix. To move forward, to try things, to find answers, to learn. Even though I was ill, I wanted to find someone who could teach me something. I needed a stranger's hands on me, to tell me everything was going to be OK. I don't know if my alternative therapies 'worked', or whether it was a placebo effect. Either way, I felt grateful for the kindness of strangers. These ongoing therapies became something I wanted to incorporate into my day-to-day life – rather than have to look for them desperately if ever I was in murky waters again.

OVER TO YOU

What alternative therapies or activities are you intrigued about?

Which would you consider trying?

Who could you connect to in your local area?

April

TO-DO LIST:

Visit my grandpa
Look at birds

Birdwatching isn't exactly something I thought I would ever do. Let alone enjoy. My husband, my mum and I went for a walk one Easter weekend in Devon and ended up doing the Topsham 'Goat Walk' – a circular route with lovely views of the Exe Estuary. As we strolled and talked and pointed at various nice houses and different types of flowers, we went past the RSPB Bowling Green Marsh Nature Reserve, a little wooden hut among the trees with a viewing platform.

There was an elderly woman there, who must have been in her nineties, wearing a forest-green fleece with a bird logo, and she was explaining to us the difference between five different types of birds (they all looked the same to us). She handed us binoculars and we nodded along, pretending to be very interested, and she spoke for a long time about these birds and how you could tell the difference between the four very similar types by the slight difference in beak shape. I remember feeling inspired: *Wow, this woman really loves this stuff. She can hardly walk, she can hardly see, and yet she is here, on a weekend, telling people in*

Spring

depth about birds. It moved me – the passion, the motivation, the simple things that get us out of bed every morning. Usually, it's as simple as doing something we love. At any age.

My grandpa suffered from dementia in the last few years of his life, and he passed away in his nineties during my year of nothing. I was gifted time with him as I wasn't working as much. He would repeat himself a lot and forget things constantly and we put a big clock next to his bed with the date and day of the week so he could root himself in some basic information, even if he needed to keep looking again and again. 'Oh, it's Monday!'

I enjoyed asking him questions about his childhood and first jobs, and he could talk to me for ages about that. He also still loved food, up until the end, which I know made my mum happy. If he loved food, that meant he still loved life, in some way.

He lived in a beautiful location in Stroud in Gloucestershire. A house made of grey Cotswold stone surrounded by flowers, it was once the bedrock of many Christmases and family gatherings. During the months before he died, we were all visiting him more often. We knew he was declining. I was of course sad at the thought of losing him but what surprised me was how sad I was at the thought of losing the house as well. The house felt like a person too, with a mood of its own; the sun always seemed to shine there, bright bluebells bloomed endlessly, and we'd pick flowers for every room and gather small, dark blackberries for pies. I became hyper-aware every time I visited the house, trying to freeze time and hold on to the memories. I went to his upstairs bathroom, and memorised the bath and the basin, which were all an old turquoise colour, and while washing my hands with a little old-fashioned bar of soap, I looked out of the window at this garden with the window slightly open and tried to breathe in the air of his house. I wanted my nostrils to always remember the warm, comforting and familiar smell. I wanted to be able to access this at any time.

My grandpa's kitchen always smelt of burning toast (from the grilling rack that would go under an Aga lid) and also Ribena. I drank a lot of strong blackcurrant cordial as a child in that kitchen. My grandma died relatively young, in her seventies, but I always remember her sitting in the kitchen in a silk robe, smoking a cigarette. There were bar stools at a window bar table, Delia Smith cookbooks, and I remember having to struggle to climb up high onto the bar stools, like they were a small mountain. When I went back recently, the bar stools looked tiny. They were the same; I had grown.

During one of the last times I visited, I kept walking past my grandpa's office and poking my head around the corner. He never went in there anymore and he slept downstairs, assisted by his carer, as he could no longer climb the stairs. His office always intrigued me – a very alive space. I remember when he used to spend a lot of time there, pottering around, listening to *The Archers*, mending something, doing admin, writing lists, organising receipts. Busy. Now, it was left just as it was, like a Tracey Emin art project, everything still in mid-flow, the lid off a pen, papers scattered across the desk, books and files left open. I always felt like I shouldn't really be looking but the door was always ajar. An invitation to pry. There was a desk with multiple drawers in front of a cork board full of documents and receipts and certificates. A desk full of stuff – lamps, vice clamps, pens, notepads, batteries, radios, sprays. A calendar on the wall, a photo of my grandma on the windowsill, a bed for late nights working where he'd sleep, endless CDs, endless books.

Spring

Before he died, my mum said I could take something. I took three books from his shelves: *How to Pray* by John Pritchard, *At the End of the Day: Enjoying life in the departure lounge* by David Winter and *In God's Hands* by Desmond Tutu. My grandpa – someone who I only ever saw as a light-hearted chappy who took pleasure in a small glass of red wine or sherry and fixed train parts and enjoyed cricket – had a whole inner life full of existential questions, prayer and faith. It made me want to go back in time and ask him more questions. When he stopped going into his office, life started to decline. It was a sign that things were going downwards. No more time or interest for hobbies. Our hobbies, no matter how small, make up so much of a life well lived.

I realise now I have a similar office space to him. I don't have a bed in there, but I do have a futon with cushions that I curl up on to hide away and read and nap. I listen to the radio. I pray. I journal. I have bookshelves. I have cabinets and receipts, postcards, trinkets, photos and a busy desk. I have things I love piled high. I have collected art and pebbles and friendship bracelets and candles, reminding me of the things and people I love. I continue my gentle yoga on the floor while I mend myself. A room of one's own. Like him.

OVER TO YOU

What is one of the most basic interests you have?

What is a small, joyful part of your day?

If you had a room of one's own, what would be in it?

What's your idea of 'pottering around' in your own company?

May

TO-DO LIST:

Cuddle a dog
Watch reality TV

I joined the BorrowMyDoggy app (which connects dog owners with local people who want to look after dogs) in May, which initially felt quite off-brand for me. Historically, I can't say I've always been a big fan of dogs. Big dogs off the lead in parks made me nervous. My dad had his hand bitten by a dog when he was younger. At my parents' villa in Portugal, there were wild dogs that would bark and show their teeth and chase you if you tried to go for a run.

My mum's side of the family had dogs growing up – a slightly hyperactive corgi called Dougal, and my grandma once had an overbred poodle that tried to bite my aunt when she was a toddler and was then taken away. My grandparents on my dad's side had a very docile dog called Sadie, who was old and soft and calm. There are pictures of me petting her when I'm two years old, offering a tennis ball.

Spring

Clearly, I do like dogs deep down. Who doesn't? They are, of course, our best friends.

I hardly watched TV before my burnout. Was never interested. I always read a book while my husband watched a film. These are our separate chosen mediums. Films are his thing – he loves the cinema and writes scripts – and books are my thing, for work and leisure. But during my burnout, my love affair with TV began. I felt like I was catching up on ten years of TV drought. I felt the need to binge on something visual and easy. I made my way through the Disney channel: *Mulan*, *Pocahontas*, *Moana*, *Encanto*. I watched all three seasons of *Motherland* in as many days. I dipped into reality TV for the first time since *The Hills* in 2006. I watched *Love Is Blind*, all seasons. *Love Island*. All I did was watch TV. All day long.

And I thought, *Well, if I'm going to be watching a lot of TV, I might as well have a companion to watch TV with me.*

I met up with people in my local area through BorrowMyDoggy. It felt like dating. I had to fill out a profile and describe myself and upload a photo. I had to get dressed properly and meet them for coffee and tell them what I do, what my lifestyle is like, what sort of person I am, and eventually they'd see my home. It felt intimate. I was on show.

First, I met up with a music producer for a coffee. He was wearing a trendy black beanie and owned a black-and-brown Dachshund puppy. I'd already looked after another Dachshund, owned by a busy young family who were always late for something. They often forget to drop off food along with the dog, so my husband and I had to improvise and buy supplies and ask around and google what to buy. My sister was shocked, said they were taking me for a ride – she paid through the nose for her dog-sitter and here I was looking after the dog for free and buying it overpriced food. The truth was,

I didn't mind at all. I actually really enjoyed the feeling of looking after the dog and pretending it was mine for a day and going through a supermarket aisle looking for nice dog food and giving it treats.

It was interesting, the process of 'matching' with dogs. I found so many gorgeous ones that slotted right in, had a relaxed temperament and clearly 'knew' I was going through something, snuggling into me and soothing my nervous system and putting their paw on my hand. Studies have shown that petting a dog or simply being in their company can reduce stress and decrease your blood pressure and heart rate. There are also studies that suggest dogs can 'sense' human sadness: be it detecting chemical changes in our sweat and breath, such as our stress hormones like cortisol, often dubbed a 'stress odour'.

I tried to look after another dog, Maisie, but she was struggling with her own mental health and didn't like men (so my husband didn't feel welcome in his own home!) and she had mood swings. As much as I could see she had a pure soul, she had a complicated back story, explained by her owner, and although I tried to make it work, her anxiety was making my anxiety worse, so I was honest and said it wasn't a good fit. I could only look after dogs that were calming and understood my situation. It felt good to be honest, to have clear boundaries. Even with borrowed dogs. And no climbing into our bed.

Dogs encouraged me to read and relax; if I reached for my laptop they would put a paw on me to stop me, or climb on top of the keyboard, wanting me to put it away. Dogs love you at your least productive. Dogs like a good walk. Dogs can watch TV with you. Dogs like a cuddle. Dogs have kind eyes. Dogs snore and breathe and eat and dream and sleep and their little heartbeat goes up and down.

OVER TO YOU

How does having pets or being around animals slow you down – or remind you of your basic needs?

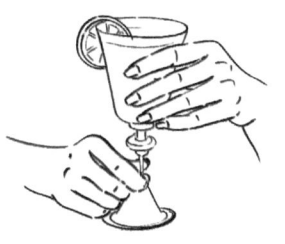

Summer

June

TO-DO LIST:

Buy crayons

Have therapy session

Being somewhat infantilised, even in adulthood, is a trait often associated with millennials. Most millennials are nearing forty by now, and yet so many have had to have help from our parents, both emotionally and financially, and we have been labelled as big snowflake babies by the media. Lots of us don't have the same financial security our parents had at our age. My dad had his university degree paid for, no debt, bought his first property in his twenties for a five-figure sum, mortgages were affordable, things were cheaper.

My parents are an incredibly stable presence in my life and always have been. My dad sits in his same chair every night, my mum buys the same newspaper every day and does her same crossword and Wordle, wearing a soft scarf and reading glasses. There's a security to this, a love that makes me feel so sheltered and safe. Routine, predictability, stability. Just as I know my husband will never leave me hanging or be late or raise his voice, my mum and dad's house is so familiar and comforting. The ideal spot for a nap is nestled in the corner of their L-shaped cream sofa, where sunlight pours in through the window. You know what to expect, and it creates a gentle hum of vibration. Now I realise that all kids really want from their parents is a feeling of safety. A quiet knowing that they love you and that they'll be there. Keeping promises. 'I'll pick you up from the station.'

In June, I ran home to my parents. I'd still failed to hand in my second novel. I'd failed to keep going with my work commitments. I'd failed to look after myself. Now I look back and can see that I was unwell, I wasn't a failure at all, but my brain was fried and my logical thinking was scrambled. My dad listened, took me seriously, and sat there with me. My mum made me tea, bought me a lovely plant, fed me home-cooked treats. My dad knows when to give me his sympathy, but he always knows when to give me a pep talk. He said to me recently: 'Keep doing what you're doing, you're doing a great job. If they don't like it, tell them to fuck off.' It reminded me of the iconic Helen Mirren quote I love: 'At seventy years old if I could give my younger self one piece of advice, it would be to use the words "fuck off" much more frequently.' Funnily enough, my therapist also told me to buy a mug that said 'fuck off' on it. Recovering burnt-out people-pleasers need visual prompts like this. Sometimes we need a gentle, nurturing environment; other times, we need a dose of tough love. One of the reasons I couldn't finish my novel is that my diary was full of annoying commitments I didn't want to do, favours for other people, 'pick-your-brain' emails I didn't have to reply to. I also have a framed piece of artwork that says 'Quiet, I'm working on my novel', which is a politer way of saying fuck off.

Spending time being back in Exeter, with my parents, was soothing. Dad was cooking lamb in the slow cooker. Mum made a lemon cake. I took myself on a day out, a nostalgic tour of Exeter, the town I used to know like the back of my hand. Virgin Megastore and HMV no longer existed: the old 'meeting places' for spending time with boys and buying VHS and CDs. Debenhams had been demolished, the place where I had my first retail job, where I wore a hideous purple shirt and hid in the changing rooms whenever boys I fancied came in. The big Topshop had gone, the place my friends and I would buy our 'going-out tops' to hit up clubs like Timepiece and Rococos. I took myself to Rougemont Gardens and saw the city through my now mid-thirty-something eyes, feeling like I was a tourist in a different world. Rougemont used to be the place I'd go on weekends with my school friends; we'd smoke rollies, get piercings, drink Lambrini, wear too much eyeliner and beads in our shoelaces and sit in a circle with random boys from the college down the road. The gardens were lush and neatly trimmed, with vibrant new flower beds in full bloom. Young families lounged nearby, enjoying picnics and ice-cream cones in the warm air.

A totally different place to what I remember from my teen years. On my walk, it felt as though I was being guided around the gardens, as if I was having a 'tour' of my memories. Something was saying: *Emma, it's time to say goodbye.* (It felt like the same guiding energy that took me around the graveyards.)

I went into Exeter Library, the place I'd studied so seriously for my A-levels with my friends. Browsing the shelves, I spotted a laminated copy of *Olive* – a full circle moment that caught me in my throat. I could remember sitting there at these tables, so vividly, revising for my exams. I wouldn't have known I'd one day find my own published novel here.

I visited the Phoenix, an arts centre that hosted various nights out when I was in my early twenties, and I sat in the corner with a decaf coffee. A song by Kansas was playing overhead: 'Carry on, my wayward son. There'll be peace when you are done.' The song is about self-encouraging, yearning, longing – the idea that life is hard and so changeable, and yet we all know there will probably be peace at the end, so keep going. I walked home through the town centre and through Fore Street, a sloping road surrounded by offbeat alleyways. Many of the old stores of my youth were no longer there, but I spotted one that hadn't closed down, called Blue Banana: a tiny haven for teen goths craving tattoos, piercings, fishnet tights, black nail polish and blue mascara. Everything was just the same – the scents, the products, the glass piercing counter. I felt like I was stepping back in time, seeing my fourteen-year-old self standing right in front of me. The girl who just wanted to fit in and be liked. Who wanted to do well at school. Who wanted to be accepted by the cool kids and would do things just to join in and be validated. I caught my reflection and instead of a teenager I saw a thirty-something woman in a scarf. *Wow. That's you. That's me. Grown-up now.* A woman who was finally learning how to take care of their inner fourteen-year-old. A deep level of shapeshifting had finally occurred.

As well as heart-to-hearts with my parents, I also received support from a woman I'll call Tilda. One coaching session with her in particular changed everything. Tilda is a friend I'd made on the Martha Beck Wayfinder coaching course. We got to know each other quite intimately via Zoom over the nine months. I saw the background of her office space every week, the roll-neck jumpers she wore, the rectangular glasses, the chin-length straightened hair. I knew about her family set-up, she knew about my imposter syndrome. I knew the little intricacies of her personality, how analytical and focused she was; she knew my biggest insecurities. In many ways, these women on the coaching course got a glimpse into a part of me that not even my closest friends had seen. Tilda was kind enough to give me mates' rates as she was still developing and practising her coaching. I felt like I was getting a good deal – she was technically a new coach, but she was a certified Enneagram teacher and had lots of experience in other areas. She was really good and a great listener.

For many social reasons, it's common to split ourselves into different versions – how we act alone, in groups, one-on-one with friends, with parents, or at work. To some extent, that's just having social skills. But for me, it felt like it had gone too far – I was performing different parts of myself instead of being whole. I wanted to feel centred again, to be one complete self.

In one particular session with Tilda, she took me through a variation on IFS Parts Therapy (Internal Family Systems). You look at the different aspects of yourself and essentially through looking at these parts, and welcoming them in, you have a chance of feeling more connected to yourself, and more aligned. Martha Beck talks a lot about the word 'integrity', from the Latin word *integer*, which literally means 'whole'. When we tap into the childlike part of ourselves, we start to heal and understand what makes us who we are. Tilda took me through an IFS session, and we spoke to the Small Emma who used to read books under the covers as a child. I realised that Performer Emma had taken over. The work-obsessed side of me was running the show and squashing the playful side of me. Performer Emma was becoming addicted to work, addicted to success. I needed the two separate sides of me to meet. I needed them to welcome and understand each other. It was so exhausting being so divided and swinging between these two identities.

It was time to nurture the child inside; she was tired and confused. She was scared of the Performer Emma, because Performer Emma didn't know when to stop and overrode her bodily signals. At my core, I am the same one Emma (obviously) but I needed to speak to all the different parts. I needed to make sense of which bits of myself were wounded, which parts could hold space for the others. After the therapy session, I felt like I no longer needed to compartmentalise myself so much. No more breaking myself down into pre-packaged pieces for other people's consumption. No more cracking the whip for the sake of it.

We change, but we also don't change. It's always healing to reconnect with the younger you. At an Elizabeth Gilbert 'Big Magic' workshop in London, she invited us to write with our non-dominant hand a letter from our child self to us now (which comes out in messy, kid handwriting). We wrote down all the things we enjoy. Here is my list:

I like to have fun

I like to eat nice food

I like to play and hug my family

I like it when I sleep and am cosy

I like it when I go outside

I like it when I make things

I like happy mornings

I like drawing and writing and swimming

I like it when you are with nice people

I like reading books

I like being in the garden

I like pens and crayons

I like a 'sick' day at home :)

At my parents' house one afternoon, we got the photo albums out and I stumbled across a photo of me as a small child, drawing at the kitchen table. I must have been about three or four. I have a big grin. Crayons all over the table. Crayons in both hands. Dark blue, stained, inky fingers. A big piece of white paper in front of me covered in drawings. *There I am*, I thought.

OVER TO YOU

What activities remind you of being a child, or bring out your childlike self?

What aspects of your eight-, fourteen-, eighteen-year-old selves do you still carry with you now?

How can you embrace your childlike, playful self more?

July

TO-DO LIST:

Burn the fleece
Wear colourful dungarees

I had been wearing the same dark-purple fleece for months without washing it.

Every morning, I got up and put this same item of clothing on, which was usually just discarded on the floor from the night before. No bra. No deodorant. Our local postman is young and good-looking and every time I answered the door with greasy hair and swinging boobs under fleece, I was mortified. And yet I couldn't be bothered to put any proper clothes on. I didn't see the point but, more critically, I didn't know who I was (yet). I was still the sluggish caterpillar. How long would this burnout last? It felt like it had been dragging on forever.

I'd text my sister, making a joke out of it, but honestly: when was I going to feel well enough to be normal again? What happened to those days of putting on a nice outfit? When would I appreciate the beautiful colours and fabrics hanging in my wardrobe? Getting dressed used to be a huge part of my enjoyment each morning. But I couldn't face wearing anything other than my jogging bottoms and this dreaded fleece. I felt like I didn't know who I was, so therefore I didn't know what to wear.

'Burn the fleece,' my sister said one day, over a cup of tea. 'And wash your hair too.'

She happened to be coming to London more frequently for work, travelling up from Bristol and staying in my spare room. I loved having her to stay, my little sis, and I've always felt that she's like a guardian angel to me, always there in my times of need, and now she was magically in my kitchen on the days when it mattered most. On one of my lowest days, she came home from work and made a cheesy pasta bake for me, reminding me of the hearty carbohydrate meals we used to eat after school. She made it with the same comforting creamy sauce that made me feel twelve again. People sometimes think she is the older sister, even though she is two and a half years younger, because she has her shit together in a way that I do not. She understands nutrition, is good at organisation, plans things meticulously. She has a Nutribullet. She tracks her sleep. She goes on long runs. She takes her vitamins. She was the perfect person to be around while I still felt wobbly about everything.

One morning, waking up feeling lethargic still, I noticed the fleece was gone. It was in the wash (I think my sister had put it there). I looked at all my clothes, none of which felt appealing. As an experiment, I felt compelled to put on the brightest item of clothing I own – a pair of rainbow dungarees. It felt like a dare. I wanted to see if it would do anything. These dungarees are loud. Primary colours. I look like a children's TV presenter in them. You cannot miss them. When I wear them out, people always assume I want to talk. That I might be a 'big personality' to be wearing such loud clothes among a sea of grey suits on the Tube. People will chat to me on public transport, or across the street. Kids will point at me and say, 'Mummy, look!' Anyway, I put them on, and they couldn't suit my mood any less. I still had an Eeyore cloud swirling above my head.

That day, I decided to book in a haircut.

My grown-out bob with split ends looked depressing. I went to my local hairdresser for a trim, wearing the dungarees. I walked in, and her eyes lit up.

'Well, well, well, I was having a properly shit day, until now! You've cheered me right up with those dungas,' she said. 'Love them.'

'You know what, I think I've cheered myself up too,' I said. I couldn't quite believe how something so trivial had the power to change my mood.

In that moment, I realised not only the power of dopamine dressing, but also the power it had to affect other people. It's like seeing a small dog on public transport, you can't help but smile. I promised myself I'd wear something fun each day for a few days to see if the experiment would stick – and it did. I bought a little figurine of the late great fashion icon Iris Apfel to put next to my bed, to remind me to have fun. Hey, like her, you never know, you might even live until you're 102. Clothes matter. Clothes are fun, and give you life. One of her catchphrases: 'More is more and less is a bore.'

This discovery reminded me of the 'change cycle', one of my favourite coaching modules in the Martha Beck course. All humans go through it. We change constantly. According to Beck, there are four squares that we go through when we face a big life-changing event like marriage, divorce, redundancy or a major birthday. It can be big or small:

Summer

> *In square one, we melt down into gloop.*
>
> *In square two, we start dreaming again and you usually make an external change (feng shui your bedroom, get a haircut, etc.)*
>
> *In square three, you put things into action. You get steadier.*
>
> *In square four, you're flying again. You have wings. The butterfly again.*

Life is constant change cycles; round and round we go. This time round, I was clearly in square two; the haircut gave it away. Even a fresh trim can represent a step forward. This was promising. I was changing a few things externally. Coco Chanel once, supposedly, said: 'A woman who cuts her hair is about to change her life.' In *Fleabag*, there is a much-loved quote, from season two: "Hair is everything!" If you see a friend who suddenly has a fringe, or bangs or a pixie cut, it's pretty likely that her life is about to change. She is different now, so give her some room to spread those new wings.

In a 2024 article penned for *Vogue*, Zadie Smith writes about her relationship with style as she ages. Reflecting on her creative life, she writes about her younger self in the third person: 'She wore only party clothes or else university sweats and pyjamas. Nothing in between. This is partly explained by the strange nature of my work, which has involved sitting alone at a home desk for the past 25 years. I was either doing that, or else going out at night, drinking and dancing.'

Like this, my wardrobe had reflected two sides of my working life: either I had very fancy clothes (patterned, well-made dresses for public events) or frayed jogging bottoms that I sat and wrote in at home, usually stained with hardened porridge. This reflected my schedule as a public and private writer. Either working like a little hermit or on a stage in front of an audience. Two extremes. Where was the middle ground? Where was I? Who was in the middle living out my day-to-day life?

C sends me links all the time to clothes I might like. *This is so YOU*, she would say, sending me a colourful dress or a jazzy jumper. Another friend sent me a picture of a mannequin with gold earrings and a patterned dress and headband, with the caption *Very Gannon*. If something is so 'me' then I must have a 'me' and a self. I just needed to find her again. This 'me' had gone missing.

Slowly, as the year went on and the summer months added some sunlight, I was moving into square three (putting things into action), finding myself again, and I decided to sell practically all my clothes. Time for some proper feng shui. I became obsessed with Vinted, an online second-hand marketplace. I sold off all my old clothes that reminded me of my former life, gave a portion to charity, and bought the brightest jumpers I could find. I loved the experience: I was buying second-hand and buying things that felt fun, typing in keywords such as 'rainbow vest' or 'chunky brogue' or 'fun pop socks'. No fast fashion or big retailers in sight. When the parcels arrived, they were wrapped nicely and smelled fresh, like flowers. I felt like I was receiving gifts, even though I had paid for them. The sellers left me notes along with the items. One woman told me the jumper I'd bought was the same one she got engaged in. Another said she'd miss the dress – it had been her lucky charm when she aced a big job interview. A third woman shared that the shoes were her favourite, but due to a foot injury she couldn't wear them anymore, and was happy they were going to a good home. These weren't just clothes on a rack – they were special pieces of someone else's life story, and they were going to help me through the next chapter of mine.

Does dopamine dressing really work? Can clothes actually give you a boost?

According to fashion psychologist Shakaila Forbes-Bell, it's less about statistics but more about our own personal associations. She said, speaking in an interview to *Harper's Bazaar* (2024): 'When we wear [certain] clothes, the associations have the power to change the way we feel and even change the way we act. So, for example, if you associate a yellow jumper with happiness, then you will embody that feeling of happiness when you wear it.'

Perhaps this was what was happening with my rainbow dungarees – they suddenly represented a choice: I was choosing to have a good day over a bad one. I was making my own associations. During my year of nothing, it was the most obvious things that I needed to remind myself of. How could I have forgotten something so simple?

Being aware of the change cycle helped me enormously. There is nothing necessarily 'wrong' with you when you're unable to live your 'best life' or have boundless energy. Sometimes, you are in the in-between. You are on ice, on pause. When we don't know who we are, we don't know what to wear, it's that simple. We are simply in square one, what Beck calls 'bug soup'. We are just the caterpillar melted down, on the way to being a butterfly again. Eventually, I found a new groove, I had changed. I was like a Pokémon, evolving. I was Emma 2.0, with a brand-new wardrobe. I was not the butterfly yet, but she was at least in sight.

OVER TO YOU

What clothes make you feel good?

Have you tried dopamine dressing?

August

TO-DO LIST:

Pack swimming costume

I never intended to get into cold water swimming. Honestly, I thought it was all a bit cliché. When I first got a copy of *At the Pond: Swimming at the Hampstead Ladies' Pond* from Daunt Books, it seemed so twee – millennial writers with their bobs and tote bags. Then I caught my reflection, bob and tote bag included, and found myself heading to the lido. (I ended up reading the book – and loving it.) Maybe it's OK to embrace a cliché, as long as you're aware of it.

It wasn't quite the Ladies' Pond, but I was headed in that direction (Parliament Hill Lido is very near the ponds). I packed my big bright-red striped bag with my swimming costume, towel dress, goggles, orange pool sliders, deodorant, mascara and hair ties. I loved people-watching at the pool. A young man was having swimming lessons; an older man in a woolly hat with his AirPods was meditating in the shallow end;

two friends swimming side by side bitching about their boss; a big burly guy in the sauna putting some lavender oil on the hot coals. Then, when I went to a friend's house for dinner, I told her about my new obsession with the lido and she showed me a huge artwork she had on the wall in her living room of that very same destination, by Jenni Murphy. The colours popped: the crystallised turquoise pool, the London city horizon behind, the green trees, the blue and red towels, the pink café sign.

It wasn't so much that I wanted to 'get into swimming' but that my body was craving being plunged into cold water. My body temperature ran hot, and I sizzled when I got in. I felt shapeless and hot and bothered and that's why I needed specifically cold water. Dipping into the iciness, I could feel myself merge with the water, a body of atoms moving through another body of atoms. It felt like the biggest relief, the water helping me shake off all my worries. When I swim, it's one of the only times I am fully in the present moment.

On a trip to Eastbourne, I was glued to the book *The Tidal Year* by Freya Bromley. I was entranced: she was finding her way back to herself via the water, after the tragic death of her beloved brother. The way she described getting into water, painting pictures of the tidal pools as being still like 'saucers of milk' – it made me want to swim, not necessarily to complete laps, but simply to immerse my restless body in an icy pool of water. It was a healing process. Bromley wrote that she would often scream under water. I wanted to try it. Swimming also became an activity that I could do with others – a way of saying: 'I'm going to be brave now, can you support me, or at least just witness it?' And, 'Shall we grab a coffee afterwards?'

As you get older, when old friends start to drift away, you realise that new friends are formed by sharing a common interest. An old friend said she moved house recently to be nearer her surfing community. Another has started playing ultimate frisbee and made a new set of friends. Another is taking up tennis lessons. Another met a new friend at a local climbing wall. Cold swimming had become my new thing, where I found that I usually ended up connecting with a certain type of woman. A woman looking for an element of bravery, or escapism, or me-time, or joy, or a fresh start. A fellow woman wearing a woolley hat, looking for a small adventure and connection.

Swimming was also a way for other people to reach out when I was ill and emotionally distant. My husband's mother and stepfather kept in touch by saying: 'Swim soon?' They live in Clacton-on-Sea, a seaside town in Essex, and occasionally we'll go for a swim in the sea. I had been honest about my burnout symptoms because I had been very distant and unable to commit to any plans. It made me feel guilty. My husband's stepfather had recently been through cancer treatment, and I felt embarrassed to be making a big deal about my burnout and cancelling plans. It was invisible and so hard to explain. But he understood, which meant a lot. Once he'd healed from his surgery, it was extra lovely when we got the chance to swim together again.

I began craving more open space, and while I loved the lido, I yearned for a larger stretch of water to swim in. Just before my breakdown I visited Jersey and my parents came with me, as I was speaking at their literary festival, the Festival of Words. We walked to the local tidal pool. They sat on the edge of the Havre Des Pas lido with their coffees and massive coats on and told me I was 'mad!' when they saw my legs, red raw from the iciness of the water. 'I can only swim in the sea on a hot holiday,' Mum said, laughing at me. There was something so intensely comforting about the two of them, sitting there, just watching me swim. I felt twelve again. Supported, watched, seen.

A few months later, my dad and I went to his local golf club for lunch. At reception, he paid for me to swim, and the act of him doing so also made me feel young again (in a nice way) – just like the Jersey trip. He showed me where the changing rooms were, and then went outside, grabbed a table, ordered a coffee and watched on in sunglasses as I swam. I'd occasionally look up and he would wave and smile. Later, he said he'd had a lovely day, how relaxing it was just sitting there, watching me swim up and down. After swimming, I was hungry and ate crisps and drank an apple juice, exactly like I used to after school.

Mum and I also went swimming in Stratford, in the big Olympic pool. She grew up near a similar-sized baths in Kent and used to go swimming there with her mother, so it all felt meaningful in the ways that small daily outings often do. The Stratford pool is well kept, the changing rooms are nice enough, and there is the Tom Daley Diving Academy, which encourages kids to dive and have fun. These gentle, slow activities made me realise all the things burnout was gifting me. Most of all: time. Leisurely activities. Things I'd not done for years, because I was too busy achieving.

For Christmas, Mum had bought me a framed picture of a woman with blonde hair and a polka-dot swimming costume going into the blue sea. It says: 'Into the water I go, to lose my mind and find my soul.' Many people might see it and find it cheesy, an Etsy print for a basic office wall, but there are moments in life where you feel very understood. Mum had noticed my new love for swimming. She'd paid attention to my new hobby and she signified it by buying me a thoughtful gift. The illustration looks a lot like me.

I always found it strange that wearing a bikini in public is basically the same as just being out and about in your underwear. I noticed that during my year of nothing my body had changed too. I always associated swimming with being young, a supple body in a stretchy bathing suit. Or being self-conscious by the pool, not wanting boys to see my body. At thirty-four, my body didn't look the same as before. I didn't mind. Older ladies showered fully nude, bushes out, smiling at you while they scrubbed their armpits. I looked at these ladies and could see my future. Learning to give less of a shit. It made me excited for the future again. *There's so much more to come,* life was saying.

OVER TO YOU

What hobbies and activities bring you utter relaxation?

What things do you enjoy, just for you, without an audience?

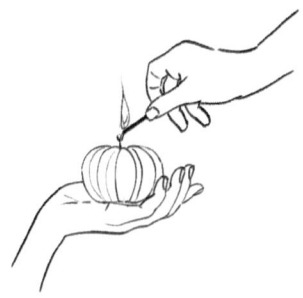

Autumn

September

TO-DO LIST:

Go on a women's-only retreat

Back in May, still piecing myself back together, I apprehensively attended a group fitness retreat. An industry contact got in touch after reading about my burnout in an essay I published on my Substack, suggesting a spot in Mallorca to eat well, work out and play games. It was a very kind gesture, but I had ignored it at first. My body was not in a state of wanting to be exerted. But once I'd rested, I took him up on the offer. I enjoyed spending time with other women who were in need of support, and not talking about work, which was a rule and really helped.

When I arrived, my room was beautiful and there was a water bottle, a cap and a welcome note on my bed. There was also an itinerary letting me know that the first exercise class of the day was at 6 a.m., starting with an ice bath. OK, this was going to be different.

I enjoyed being around other people and having our meals cooked, but I was still feeling slightly removed from life. My dissociative symptoms were coming back. The sun burned in the sky without a name, just a hot ball of fire. Trees felt upside down, and the names and faces of the new people I met danced around and I kept getting people confused. In hindsight, I think I was seeing the world through fresh eyes again. Like a newborn who doesn't have a name yet. Everything seemed new and strange, as if I were dreaming.

After that trip, I realised something was missing. Physical exercise and plant-based foods are great when getting back on your feet, and I had an enjoyable time in the sunshine – but I also knew it was a stepping stone towards something deeper. I could not care less about having toned abs or doing a record number of burpees. I like moving and swimming, but I'm more likely to watch a Joe Wicks workout in bed while eating toast than choose to do a solo HIIT workout. I wanted to find something that was more focused on spirituality and connection. I wanted to go further inwards. I wanted to find a place to retreat in stillness and silence. A recommended, legitimate one too – without anyone preaching or reading me sermons or selling me £100 crystals. I wanted a community who could help me explore a solid, rooted, spiritual practice. Then I found myself magnetically drawn towards intuitive healer Fiona Arrigo.

Cut to September: did I think, on my outbound flight to Malaga from Gatwick Airport, that a few days later I would find myself skinny-dipping with two women I'd just met, in a big pool overlooking the Andalusian mountains, howling like wolves at the full moon? No, I did not.

I discovered Fiona Arrigo's retreat via a friend who found her online community transformative. The retreat was focused on 'deep rest'. I assumed I was going to have a week of walks, dinners and rest, as this was what was billed on the itinerary. I didn't realise just how that would feel in my body, or how much it would positively impact my overall frame of mind, long after I returned to London (where the man next to me on my flight home ate crisps aggressively loudly – just to test me, I'm sure).

The retreat was held in the Spanish town of Gaucín, in a charming finca with a turquoise pool and mountain views. The sun was strong and the rooms were clean, simple and elegant. We ate three meals a day together on a beautiful long wooden table outside. The incredible chefs nourished us and would garnish our desserts with edible flowers and tie fresh lavender stems to our napkins.

Every morning we had a workshop with Fiona, which involved sitting in a circle, lighting natural incense, playing soft music, being still, listening and being open to sharing if you felt called to. In the first introductory women's circle, I felt my palms go sweaty. We went round the circle and each shared our story, our family lineage, where we're at, what we want from life. I don't get nervous anymore when I do any public speaking on stage to do with my work – but this felt different. This was a bunch of kind faces ready to receive whatever you wanted to share. I clammed up and my throat closed over. I shared a recent family loss, my burnout experience and where I am now. No one pandered, no one rubbed my arm, there were no overt facial expressions apart from a brief nod. *Oh*, I thought, *I get it*. I get it. This is about the power of simply sharing in a safe space. There was a relief in this understanding. It was surprisingly moving. I didn't want to be hugged, I just wanted to share something, out loud, in a welcoming space.

Fiona repeated these same words many times over the course of the week: 'When women come together, they heal.' When she first said them during our first women's circle, I wasn't sure I needed healing. By day six, I realised what she meant. We'd had morning women's circles, meditation time with delicious natural candle scents floating through the air, sound baths, and we even made friendship bracelets together. Underneath the outer exterior of all these women was something similar and familiar in all of us. Worries, relationship rifts, self-blame, unprocessed stories, fear of the unknown. There were no burdens being cast, no one was asked to carry anything for anyone else, we were simply sharing – it felt freeing. I found myself sleeping more intensely, having very vivid dreams and breathing more deeply. I shared a room with a friend (the same friend who had recommended the retreat) and each night we fell asleep giggling about something that had happened that day. It reminded me of being at a sleepover as a young girl.

During the week, I saw just how positively my nervous system responded to the company of women. Perhaps it was the softly spoken voices, the panoramic views of green foliage, the genuine compliments ('I love your clothes/tattoos/earrings') and just the act of being really sweet and kind to each other. This isn't to reduce or caricature women – we are not all sunlight and whispers and braiding each other's hair – but there was something beautiful about this specific group and how we gelled; it was all just really gentle. It was like we'd all arrived in a box labelled 'Handle with care'. Something that feels counter-cultural in the harsh world we live in. (We all absolutely agreed that men need this work too.)

There was heaps of time to do nothing. In the afternoons, everywhere you looked someone was having a nap on a sofa or sun-lounger. This was so refreshing in a culture of to-do lists. Most afternoons after our various activities, we took our journals and lay by the pool. I am usually the odd one out in my family or friendship group – constantly journalling, reading, daydreaming, thinking up stories, staring at the moon. And now here I was with a group of women who all did the same introspection as me. In the words of Marina Keegan: 'We don't have a word for the opposite of loneliness' – but that's how it felt. I felt the opposite of lonely.

In terms of activities, it was all really soft and slow: we moved our bodies (I love the word 'movement' much more than 'exercise'), one evening we enjoyed making crafts together, finding joy in creating with our own hands. I made a bookmark by threading bits of cotton. We set out on silent morning hikes, soaking in the landscape bathed in warm orange light. We did Pilates by the pool. We had breathwork sessions and I had a one-to-one session with Fiona, surrounded by brightly coloured foliage like wild poppies and lavender. We had a 'closing' ceremony, which I loved: a chance to sew myself back up before going home.

Retreats are not cheap. Every tiny weeny thing is lovingly prepared and thought about, down to the silk sleep mask on your pillow, and thus, it is not real life. It is often marketed to you as 'an investment'. When in a perfect environment like this, there is often a creeping thought in the back of your head that cranks up, along these lines: 'What if I could live like this FOREVER? What if I sell my house and buy some chickens and move to the mountains? I could live simply. I could only have two sets of clothes! Then I would have ZERO worries.' But this isn't the point of a retreat, at least not for me. I like my city life. I don't want to eliminate all noise, challenges or variety. I just want more tools to help me move through it. Retreats are a chance to look at yourself, reflect and make changes, but it does not mean needing to overhaul every crevice of your being overnight, take an axe to your relationships or light a match to everything and anything. For me, this trip was a reminder that I can stay calm even in rush hour, if I choose to. This was not about changing the outside structures right now, but about tuning in to the layers underneath, changing up the insides. The frequencies of my life. Adding in more beauty and trust. If I could share two words that summed up my experience of the retreat, it would be these: magic and medicine.

My personal learnings felt deeper, calmer and more potent. I wasn't sitting at the front of class with my journal like I was in my twenties, hoping a 'guru' might save me. I wasn't looking to be taught anything new. I wasn't looking for answers. I wanted someone to help me discern and peel things away. I was looking for an opportunity to take things off my pile, not add anything new on.

It was like a collective hand-on-heart moment: I will no longer harm myself. By harming myself, I am harming the planet. I will no longer punish myself by over-working, over-giving, over-thinking or over-doing it. I know myself now. I know what feels good and what feels uncomfortable. This retreat reminded me that this peace and stillness does exist. It can exist. It filled me with the biggest sense of hope and possibility during a time of massive change and troubling realities. It was a reminder to trust myself and steer my own ship as best I can. A reminder to look around you. If nothing else, nearby there will most certainly be a beautiful flower. Start there.

OVER TO YOU

What does deep rest look or sound like to you?

Have you been intrigued about investing in a retreat?

How can you incorporate these still moments in your everyday life?

October

TO-DO LIST:

Drink less alcohol
Drink more water

It was October and I decided to give up booze. I'd been drinking less in general, but then would still have nights where I'd notice I was numbing myself. My husband took me for a beautiful dinner and wine pairing and I realised that the wine had ruined the meal because I wasn't able to taste the food. I was getting progressively more drunk with each course, and the next day I couldn't remember what we'd eaten or what we'd really spoken about. Is that how I wanted to celebrate a birthday, the passing of time, the privilege of getting older? I didn't want to be drunk when I'm having dinner (especially with someone I love), I wanted to be with him, see him, listen to him. I wanted to make sure the memories were clear and not fuzzy. I wanted to put the habit away, for good.

Earlier in the summer, I'd also gone for lunch with two friends. The rosé was flowing, and when I got home I realised that I didn't have fun. Did any of us really have anything in common now, apart from a few things from the past? Would we have much to talk about, without the free flowing of the sugary wine? I was going through life on cruise control with alcohol greasing the wheels, but I wasn't really making any conscious or empowering decisions. The alcohol had to go. I needed to clear the decks to understand what was truthful underneath. And I needed to work out what I wanted and who I was, underneath the fuzz of a chemical blanket.

Like many millennials who grew up in a smallish town, my relationship with alcohol came barrelling into my life hard and fast. Teens getting their stomach pumped on the weekend was a pretty normal occurrence; so was giving a stranger on the street a tenner to buy you and your mates a bottle of cheap vodka. 'She's speaking on the big white telephone' was slang in Devon for having your head down the toilet (while being physically and metaphorically sick on spirits).

Everyone found it funny back then: funny that one time I woke up in a flower bed, and that none of us could ever remember getting home. On holiday in Spain aged sixteen, I got so sick on sangria that, let's just say, I never drank anything 'with bits in' ever again. Then, university happened, and those three years went by in a white-wine blur. Cheap trebles, bright-blue shots, the snakebite concoction of lager, cider and blackcurrant. Constant low-hum headaches and empty bottles rattling about under the bed. Entering the world of work, with 'after-work drinks', where you got to find out all the juicy stuff about your colleagues and your boss. I drank my way through all those nights too, without ever stopping to ask: is there an option *not* to do this?

It took me ages to unpick my relationship with drinking. My career was gaining momentum and in my spare time I was reading self-help books and watching TED Talks. Through my job as the host of a podcast, I was interviewing psychologists, therapists, experts talking about mental health and listening to doctors explaining facts about our diet, brain chemistry and behavioural patterns, but the elephant in the room was the fact that I was still drinking every night.

I really wanted to change my relationship with alcohol and started making progress. Then, 2020 happened. Even Gwyneth Paltrow admitted to knocking back the whisky sours seven nights a week during the first national lockdowns due to Covid-19. And if it was good enough for the founder of a global wellness brand, it was good enough for me. I made a playlist to get drunkenly emotional to. I purchased things while drunk. I bought tickets to a band I used to like when I was younger and then asked for a refund when I'd sobered up. I sent people sentimental text messages, waking up the next day wincing. Nothing that bad happened, but I was drinking more and more again each night, convincing myself it was nothing but a chic wind-down part of my routine. I remember placing a huge wine order, thinking it was fine because it was organic, with a trendy east-London label on it. But I was taking a big bag of clinking bottles out to the recycling bin every week. Something occasional had slowly turned into a nightly habit again, and I couldn't pinpoint when.

It was only when I interviewed author Ruby Warrington, who coined the term 'sober curious', that things started to really change. Ironically, I'd arrived at the interview severely hungover, but Ruby's non-judgemental message of turning a curious eye to your drinking habits, and/or the role drinking plays in society, got my attention. After yet another lockdown was announced, I sheepishly got her book down from my bookshelf (*Sober Curious: The Blissful Sleep, Greater Focus, Limitless Presence, and Deep Connection Awaiting Us All on the Other Side of Alcohol*). With a deep breath, I decided to be genuinely curious, and admit I really wanted something to seriously change.

Some people have to give up drinking completely; they can't have a couple because they know where it would lead. Addiction is real. It requires a serious, courageous ongoing recovery process. That feels separate to what I'm describing here. I had fallen into grey-area drinking, reminiscent of a phrase created by life coach Jolene Park, who says you don't necessarily have a 'drinking problem'; instead, you have a 'problem with drinking' without it being a severe alcohol-use disorder.

Many of us want to question our relationship with alcohol while also maintaining the possibility of moderation. The insidious involvement of drink in our daily lives means that until you reach rock bottom there has been little incentive to question it as a lifestyle choice, until recent years. My question is: why do we have to wait until we have a serious problem to question our habits? I wanted to give up getting drunk. There was nuance to the conversation for me, and it wasn't until I discovered the mindful drinking movement that I felt I could put words to this without needing to label myself.

Without alcohol, I found myself reconnecting to the part of myself that didn't need to binge or fill a hole. I reconnected with my body and learnt how to settle my nervous system through breathwork. I started being more honest with my loved ones, I made changes in my career, I stopped people-pleasing. I found space in my life to be creative for the sake of it. I committed to journalling. I no longer wanted to numb myself out.

Now, I have alcohol-free beers in the fridge, because I prefer them. I don't miss getting drunk at all. I wake up earlier, have fewer headaches, and feel more present in my day-to-day life. To me, being sober-curious is about living with intention rather than going through the motions. Some friendships faded – those built on nothing more than drinking or drunken gossip have drifted away. I don't get invited to crazy parties anymore. I'm better for it.

OVER TO YOU

Are you intrigued by the term sober-curious?

Are you curious about your relationship with alcohol?

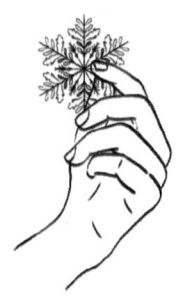

Winter

November

TO-DO LIST:

*Write a letter to your
future self*

Nearly a year after the New Forest meltdown incident, I went away with the same friend, C, who'd witnessed it. We went to a cabin in Suffolk this time, a place we'd stayed at years ago – so we were familiar with the set-up and came prepared, stocking up on bread, milk, Camembert and fruit beforehand. We've known each other since we were four years old and we have that type of honesty where we're more like sisters. We love each other, we can share a bed no problem, but we can also squabble. She has a tendency to try to fix things (like we all do) and sometimes her maternal nature can feel slightly suffocating. On the drive to the cabin, we spoke about the New Forest situation and I told her the truth.

'You were trying to help too much,' I said, remembering how she was frantically trying to run me a bath when I was having a panic attack. In hindsight, it had made things worse.

I wanted to run my own bath and close the door. I didn't want anyone making a fuss – it only heightened the sense that something was really wrong.

In the cabin, we lit the fire and cosied up under the thick blanket with mugs of tea and started chatting about all sorts of things. We were clearing the air, and feeling closer because of it.

'You seem different. You're not shying away from things as much. You're being more honest,' she said.

'What do you mean?'

'You're able to talk about sad things. You used to never want to go there.'

She was right, I was able to lean further into the discomfort: the truth, the sadness, the realities of a changing life, in a way I didn't do before. I wasn't shutting things out as much. I did feel changed; it was like I could breathe again, like I had capacity in my lungs, heart and head.

'Isn't it funny,' I said to C, as we both nodded off to sleep, 'that when we go to bed at night, we don't have to do anything. Our bodies breathe for us, our heart beats for us. We just have to lie there. Not really doing anything.'

'Mmmm,' she said, drifting off, the moon shining so brightly through the skylight in the ceiling. So bright that I could see a smiling face made by craters. Things had changed, and I was starting to feel better after such a strange year. Our friendship had weathered some rocky currents, and now it rested like a ship, safely moored.

✳ ✳ ✳

My year of nothing allowed me time to embrace the mysteries of life. I didn't have answers – no clear reason for the burnout, no tidy explanation for why I felt the way I did. All I knew was that, in the moment, I managed to steer myself towards safety. It was starting to look a little bit like 'faith'. I remember a few years ago, sitting on a bench in a park in Wanstead with my husband, wondering where my creativity comes from. The mystery of it all used to spook me:

'I write all these books, but I don't feel like they come from me, necessarily. I don't understand it.'

'Where do you think they come from?' he asked.

'I don't know.'

'Maybe, one day, you will know.'

'Or, maybe I won't.'

'Yes, maybe you won't.'

It all felt like a big mystery. The words spilling out of my finger tips. The stories I needed to tell. I guess that's the point of life. We don't really *know* anything. This need to write, the countless ideas that float into my brain and become realised on the page. I often find myself wondering where I'm 'downloading' all of this from, or where we came from, where life itself originates. It's one of the oldest questions of humankind. And there I was, thinking I could solve it over a quick coffee on a Sunday afternoon with my husband.

❄ ❄ ❄

I read a lot of books during my year of nothing. I remember reading Suleika Jaouad's book *Between Two Kingdoms*, about her journey with leukaemia and survival and creativity, and became so entranced by her. I listened to countless interviews, typing her name into my podcast app, listening to her talk about how creativity itself is an act of survival. I had also been writing myself letters from unconditional love – a practice I'd learnt from my friend Selina (who describes it as downloading advice from 'your wise older self') and also Elizabeth Gilbert, who runs the 'Letters From Love' newsletter on Substack.

A few months later, Elizabeth Gilbert herself got in touch, asking me if I would write a Letter From Love for her Substack community. It was such an honour to be asked. You write the prompt 'Dear Love, what would you have me know today?' And you take your pen, and you wait for a response, and you write it down.

A year to the day that I had my full burnout meltdown (23 October 2022), the day I lay in bed not knowing if I would ever feel alive again, my Letter From Love was published on Elizabeth Gilbert's newsletter (23 October 2023). Coincidence?

> *Dear Love, what would you have me know today? Oh, sweet teary one – I totally get it, I do. You are so worried, so worried about what is going on in the world and worried about the struggles of those you love. Let me sit with you while you sob. Let me witness those warm tears that land on your cheeks and let me do nothing with them, for they don't need to go away or be fixed. Just let them land.*
>
> *I'm here, just as I always am, writing through your hand. Have you noticed that I have always been here, since the day you could write and breathe and feel and be? All you need to do is call on me and I will be here.*
>
> *Oh, my angel – the world is a lot, isn't it? And you feel so much of it. Let it move through you. This is normal, this is the natural way of things, and I am here.*
>
> *I'm here to listen, to be still, to watch and to be with you. I will always love you and I will always be here*

whenever you need to cry. You can cry with me whenever you want. You can always come to me.

Promise me a swim tomorrow? Or a small walk? Maybe go to the tea hut and see the ducks? See the beauty. See your own beauty. You've got this, you are strong, but you also need to replenish.

Go and see some lovely things. There is no one to impress.

I love you.

I realised that in the worst of my burnout I had already been writing myself letters from love, I just hadn't been calling it that, officially. On one of the worst days, I would grab my journal, and my hand would write loving things to me. Were they coming from me? Or my dead relatives? Or 'God'? Or what?

I wrote myself a letter on perfectionism:

Dear Emma,
You want to know why you can't just live in a constant state of bliss and perfection. You don't like that word 'perfection' because you don't think you are a perfectionist because you write quickly and freely. You don't mind typos, so you can't be a perfectionist! But you are being a perfectionist in many aspects of your life. You want the perfect life, you want to have made the perfect choices, you want the perfect career. You don't like that you're ill right now, it's ruining your perfect holiday.

My love, you know it can't be this way – you know that, deep down. I love the messy, imperfect parts of you. I think it's time to let go of perfection and just embrace this journey you're on.

Keep travelling, my little traveller. I love you. Be imperfect.

Then, I wrote myself a letter about the jealousy I felt about someone who'd haunted me for years.

> *Dearest Emma,*
>
> *You wanted to ask me about jealousy and X's success. You wanted to ask me about why this jealousy has haunted you since 2018. Well, my love, I think you know what I'm about to say: she is a teacher. Whether you like it or not, she is teaching you something – how to ultimately let go and lean into yourself. Your life is for living, not hers. She is on her path and guess what? It's not your path. It's got nothing to do with you. You watch it closely, because you want what she has. But what do you really want? I think you want to live with more gusto, you want to eat and indulge and enjoy and delve into life like she does. And guess what? YOU CAN! You can. It's all for the taking, and you will continue growing. You will have your own version, you already do. Emma, I PROMISE you, your life is just as delicious. It is yours and it is sacred and she is only teaching you to look at your life.*
>
> *Until next time, I love you.*

Looking back over my letters and journals during my year of nothing, I am reminded that although it was difficult and strange and I was unmoored, there was a friendly, loving presence there at all times.

I was being guided all along; I wasn't alone.

OVER TO YOU

Can you write yourself a letter from love, today?
(Even if you think it's cheesy.)

December

TO-DO LIST:

Acceptance

Carry on journalling

The word 'breakdown' has negative connotations, but I actually quite like it. I also like the word 'meltdown'. It makes me think of a caterpillar melting or breaking down inside a cocoon. I like the words 'shapeshift' and 'morph' too. It reminds me of nature – things in nature are always changing, mutating, evolving, transforming. There are so many other descriptive words we can use to describe these periods in life: nervous breakdown, collapse, fatigue, exhaustion, depletion. We can also call it 'existential burnout'. Essentially, this kind of breakdown is a way of life saying to you: this current way you are living isn't working, and it can happen at any age. Time to transform – but not without some pain.

In nature, things are allowed to break down and regenerate and build back up again. 'Going Underground' by The Jam is one of my dad's favourite songs.

In her infamous 2021 Emmy Awards speech, writer and actor Michaela Coel said: 'Do not be afraid to disappear –

from it, from us – for a while, and see what comes to you in the silence.' In premise, it's great advice. In reality: it's terrifying. Going underground is the closest we come to experiencing our own death – our deep fears rearing their dramatic head. If I go away for a bit, will anyone miss me? What if nobody notices I'm gone at all? Turns out, when you face your fears, you really do grow a new skin afterwards.

There are other ways of describing this subterranean period in culture or in conversation:

Being 'in the soil' (transforming underground).

Having a 'fallow year' (a farmer not growing any crops for a while so that the quality of the soil can eventually improve).

Living in 'the liminal space', from the Latin limen, *which means 'threshold'. Limbo comes from the Middle English lymboa: 'A place where innocent souls exist temporarily until they can enter heaven'.*

Even though we understand deep down that these phases in life are temporary, the uncertainty of not knowing when they'll end – or when we'll be ready to move forward – can be truly bewildering. It's that *'insert here'* kind of feeling: a blank page, the great unknown.

Some people call it an old-fashioned existential crisis; apparently we're due one every five to ten years. Or a quarter-life/mid-life crisis, depending on your age. Researcher and storyteller Dr Brené Brown calls it 'the mid-life unravelling': when the armour that you've built up over your teens and twenties comes crumbling down. Some people refer to it as the 'cocoon period' or a bear hibernating for the winter, sinking into a state of torpor, to ultimately conserve energy. It's a vortex of some kind, or a gateway. Writer Anne Helen Petersen refers to these life transitions as 'The Portal', describing this strange period as 'painful and discombobulating'. Author Sam Baker calls it 'The Shift', particularly in relation to women growing older, with changing bodies. Back in the day, Britney Spears hinted at this liminal space in her song 'I'm Not a Girl, Not Yet a Woman'. Therapist Donna Lancaster recently coined the phrase 'menoportal' to describe the menopause – a natural biological transition that we still don't know enough about. There are so many different types of liminal portals (temporary housing, pregnancy, maternity leave, career garden leave) whereby lots of emotions and fears arise: we have no idea what's going to happen next, and it's something we are uncomfortable with. Our identity doesn't feel solid. I was saying goodbye to my former self.

There is a Dutch word, *niksen*. It means doing nothing, or letting go, or stopping. Olga Mecking, the author of *Niksen: Embracing the Dutch Art of Doing Nothing* describes it as 'letting go of the outcome'.

I suppose it doesn't really matter what you call it, which is why I've decided to brand my particular flavour of liminal meltdown 'a year of nothing'. I felt like a ghost, floating, untethered (as I mentioned earlier, I visited graveyards more than I ever have before). People sometimes say 'I didn't really feel like I was there' during intense life transitions, and that is exactly how I felt. I didn't feel 3D, I had to literally 'ground myself' and 'find my roots' – something I've heard many yoga instructors over the years say and never really listened to or understood.

We all have to grieve losses: family losses, identity loss, career loss – and on a bigger scale: climate change and grieving the mess of the planet and the loss of wildlife. My youthful, jovial personality was shedding like a snake, my vision was cloudy and narrow. My voice sounded different. I felt like I was shifting up a gear. The young maiden becomes a crone.

As a writer who is used to working solidly and always jotting things down, I kept a diary throughout this year of nothing, which eventually turned into this book you're reading now.

So, this is my thank-you letter to my year of nothing—*

*—that turned out to be everything.

Afterword

When people ask how my burnout felt, I always say: inevitable. The ever-changing metamorphosis of us all. Even though it was scary and horrible at the time, it also felt deeply necessary. I'd been heading towards it, slowly, for years, so when the breakdown moment happened, it almost felt like a big relief. It's called a 'tipping point' for a reason. Like a bucket of water.

In the documentary *American Symphony* (2023), the Grammy award-winning musician Jon Batiste says:

> *What we love about music is that it sounds inevitable. It's playing the thing that we all know is unfolding, whether we want to accept it or not.*

Life, like music, is always unfolding, like a great symphony. After publishing countless books, tuning out my emotions, numbing occasionally with alcohol and being glued to my phone for so long, something had to give. My real life and inner essence were being ignored and clearly wanted to be noticed. Someone once told me that 'capacity' is our superpower. And when anything runs out of capacity (a bridge, an internet connection, a human brain), it breaks. Having capacity and a sense of expansiveness is a true sign that we are doing well.

Although I'm better now and my year of nothing feels at a distance from life, I want to remember the elements of the year that felt gooey like vanilla pudding. Slowing down felt truly delicious at times. Even though my brain wasn't working as normal, I was allowing myself to rest after years of being so uptight, and it felt like melting into a mound of warm butter. That feeling of your head hitting a soft marshmallow of a pillow. The enjoyment of sinking into a day-time nap. Drawing a warm evening bath with a soft-pink sky glowing outside.

As I write this, it's 2024 and it's turned out to be my year of travel. I've just returned from visiting a friend in Lisbon. I've been in Brussels on a writing trip. I spent New Year in Vietnam with my husband. I am preparing for another swim session this time at Guernsey Literary Festival and book events this year are taking me to New York. My approach to people and life has changed so much since last year – it still surprises me how different things feel. On the outside, things may not seem that different, but on the inside, it's as though a lens has been changed on a camera. I see things differently. I'm stronger, less fragile, less afraid. When you are deep in the thick of burnout and recovery, you really don't think you'll ever be well again. And then it passes, just like everyone says it will. You realise the power of you're own resilience, and you have a toolbelt that feels rightfully earned.

• • •

So here are five lessons I will take forward with me, from my year of nothing:

Afterword

LESSON 1

Prioritise those you love. Whenever I find myself getting into a tailspin about something, I remember everything I learnt about pausing, reflecting, taking a minute, choosing a different way, changing the tune. After a stressful work period, I booked off a week and visited my parents, family or friends. I looked up a place to cold swim and my dad and I went on a day trip to Firestone Bay. Remember how special the small things are. Make time for it.

LESSON 2

Gather trinkets. The little ornaments, physical items, gifts and symbols really helped me during the hard times. I have a cherubic angel figurine from Lladró on my desk from my grandpa's house, alongside an angel decoration bought by my mum in New York, plus a tortoise to remind me to go slow, and a marble elephant from my recent trip to Vietnam that symbolises good health. Keep your reminders close.

LESSON 3

Keep on top of things. Face things, don't hide them away. Clear out physical stuff, look at the monsters under the bed; don't hoard too much, clean things out regularly. Have the difficult conversation, don't let it fester or lurk. When we really look at the stuff building in our cupboards, we are subconsciously looking at the 'stuff' in our lives too.

LESSON 4

Listen to your body. Tune in to the parts of yourself that are needing love and attention. Don't forget how wise it is, wiser than our frantic minds. Grab a copy of Louise

Hay's Heal Your Body. *If in doubt, stretch. Rotate your hips in a circular motion. Find some grass and touch it with your bare feet.*

LESSON 5

You have time. *It might feel like you have to rush, move forward, make quick decisions, go, go, go. But you really do have time. Slow down. You don't need to rush. Take five. Grab a cup of tea. It's going to be OK. Breathe.*

I certainly feel more robust now: so far away from the woman who couldn't even go downstairs and make a slice of toast.

During our recent trip to Vietnam, my husband and I went on a hike together. We went slightly off-piste by accident. We had declined the offer of a tour guide (whoops) and found ourselves going downhill through a track that was getting narrower and narrower and harder to navigate. He kept slipping on mud and falling over, and I tried hard not to do the same. We were holding on to pieces of strong bamboo in order to help us navigate down the side of the muddy mountain. It was precarious. We could see that there were huts in the distance, through some of the trees, and we knew we just needed to get down to ground level. It was only 1 p.m., so lots of daylight still and we weren't in danger of it getting dark just yet. But I was starting to feel slightly nervous in the pit of my stomach. What if we got lost? Trapped? What if one of us hurt ourselves? I held it together, taking each small step. I didn't act scared, or say anything negative, I just got on with trying to get us down safely. My husband was leading the way well.

When we eventually reached the bottom, we found a river. On the opposite bank we could see there was a small village, where people were outside their houses sweeping their gardens.

Afterword

The problem was, there was no way to cross. We couldn't find a series of small rocks that would get us to the other side safely. Instead, we started climbing around bigger rocks, holding on for dear life, before realising they were too slippery and we might fall. Then, I decided to just take off my shoes and started wading through the rushing river.

We had to do something. My husband was waiting on a rock, still trying to suss out a way to go without taking off his boots. I was already out of the water, waving at him, feet sopping wet, wringing out my socks, telling him to just do it, and he did.

We saw a couple with a tour guide in front of us, so with our wet feet, we followed them for a bit around boggy rice paddies, and then eventually found ourselves at an amazing café in the sky with the most beautiful views I've ever seen. We dried out our clothes, socks and boots in the warm sunshine, and ordered a cold drink. A beautiful red butterfly landed on my hand. It was hard not to see that as a positive sign. I was stronger now. We'd made it through a tough stretch, and now we were reaping the rewards.

Back in London, when I returned to have a reflexology session with Isabel, it had been over a year since my breakdown moment with her. She greeted me in reception, and we hugged. I lay down on the massage bed, the same music playing on a loop, the same pink flowers on the wallpaper, the same tranquil energy. The room was exactly the same. I was totally different.

'You look very nice. I am happy,' she nodded, dimming down the lights and closing the door while I changed.

After the reflexology session, I asked her what she sensed. Anything? *What did you find?* I wanted to know. My feet were slippery with lavender oil, and I sipped on a cup of cold water she brought me. She said nothing – just nodded and kept on smiling at me.

Acknowledgements

Thank you so much to JP Watson, genius mind behind the Pound Project where *A Year of Nothing* was originally born. It was a difficult time in my life, but it brought such a fruitful creative project, and it really proved to me that I can write in whatever situation I'm put in. That makes me proud to be a writer, and to have such a supportive creative community around me.

The original books were first published in a smaller format, as a set of two. They also came with joyful illustrations by Georgia-Maia, who I'll always be grateful for as she designed the cover too, with a beautiful tree representing the different seasons.

Thank you to the team at Whitefox Publishing (Hannah Bickerton, Julia Koppitz, John Bond, Kiana Palombo) and Jenni Davis, Vaidehi Tikekar and Holly Kyte. Thank you to Anna Morrison for designing my cover of dreams. It's been really fun working with you to bring this new version to life and in a different way.

Thank you to my readers of 'The Hyphen' on Substack (thehyphen.substack.com) – you've kept me going.

Thank you to my mentor and guide Julia Cameron and for being the first reader of this book and writing the foreword for it.

Thank you to Betty and Ursula, the mini Dachshunds who kept me company on the sofa.

Thank you, Mum, Dad, Jo and Charlotte.

Thank you, Paul, for building our beautiful home, garden and life together. Thank you to all my friends and family for living through my year of nothing with me. I love you.

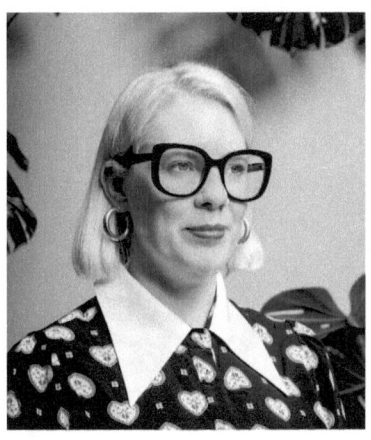

Emma Gannon is the *Sunday Times* bestselling author of eight books, including *A Year of Nothing* and *Olive*, her debut novel, which was nominated for the Dublin Literary Award. Her second novel, *Table for One*, published in 2025 with HarperCollins. Emma also runs the popular Substack newsletter 'The Hyphen', which has thousands of paid subscribers. She also hosts creativity retreats all over the world and was a judge for the 2025 Women's Prize for Non-Fiction. She is the author of the forthcoming *A Creative Compass*, to be published by Transworld, Penguin.

www.ingramcontent.com/pod-product-compliance
Lightning Source LLC
Chambersburg PA
CBHW060456080526
44584CB00015B/1450